How to optimize your fertility and get pregnant naturally...(and what to do if it doesn't happen)

Copyright 2013 by Pregnancy Bible

Jessica Randolph

All rights reserved worldwide. No part of this book may be reproduced, replicated, redistributed, stored in a retrieval system, given away or transmitted in any form or by any other means, electronic, photocopy or otherwise without the prior written permission of the publisher.

This book is for your personal enjoyment and education only. It is a general health related informational product. As an express condition of reading the book you agree to the following terms:

The content of this book is not a substitute for direct, personal or professional medical advice or diagnosis. None of the treatments, remedies or recommendations should be followed without consultation with a registered and reputable physician or health care provider. There are risks associated with actively practicing the activities and/or advice mentioned in this book for people in poor health or pre-existing physical conditions. Should you choose to use advice in this book, you do so of your own free will and accord.

Under no circumstances including but not limited to negligence shall the copyright owner be liable for any special or consequential damages that result from the use of or the inability to use this book, even if the owner has been advised of the possibility of such damages.

You agree to hold the owner of this book, the agents coauthors, contributors and employees harmless from any and all liability for all claims for damages due to injuries, including attorney fees and costs incurred by you or caused to third parties by you arising out of the products, services and activities discussed in this book. Facts and information are believed to be accurate at the time of writing this book. All data provided in this book is to be used for informational purposes only. Information provided is not all-inclusive and is limited to information that is made available and such information should not be relied upon as all inclusive or accurate.

If you do not agree with these terms and express conditions, DO NOT READ THIS BOOK. Your use of this book and any participation in the activities mentioned means you are agreeing to be legally bound by these terms.

If you would like to share this book with another person, please purchase an additional copy for each recipient. If you are reading this book and did not purchase it, or it was not purchase exclusively for you please return to the site you purchased this copy from and purchase your own copy. Please respect the hard work of the author.

Table of Contents

Introduction 6
Chapter 1 What To Do Before You Start Trying 11
    Six Months Before Conception 11
    Will The Odd Cigarette Cause Any Harm? 12
    Surely Caffeine Is OK? I Need My Coffee To Function! 12
    What About Alcohol? 12
    Does Sleep Affect Fertility? 12
    Coming Off Birth Control 13
    Are Environmental Hazards Relevant To Me? 13
    How Much Exercise Is Healthy When I Am Trying For A Baby? 13
    How Important Is Body Weight? 14
    What Foods Are Most Important In My Pre Conception Diet? 14
Chapter 2: Back To School: Important Lessons In Reproductive Health (this will contain at least five things you did not know!) 16
    Is infertility increasing? 16
    The Technical Bit: The Four Primary Reproductive Hormones 16
    What Happens At Conception? 17
    The Three Primary Fertility Signs (Get to know these well and you may save yourself thousands of dollars in unnecessary tests) 18
    Why should I chart my temperature after I am pregnant? 21
        What if there is no cervical mucus? 22
    Secondary fertility signs 23
        What a hassle! 23
        But What If I Have Irregular Cycles? 24
Chapter 3 Age and Fertility. Phew! Not As Scary As I Thought 25
    Why women are delaying pregnancy until their 30s 26
    The psychology of trying to get pregnant 27
    Nurture your relationship with your partner 28
        Remember to make love, not just have sex 28
Chapter 4 Will Anything I Do Adversely Affect My Fertility? 30
    Will Excessive Stress Affect My Fertility? 30
    Will Depression Affect My Fertility? 31
    Why are some women more fertile than others? 31

Chapter 5 Male Fertility 32

Help! We have a sperm issue- What can be done? 32

Supplements for low sperm count 33

Hormonal treatments 33

Hi Tech treatments 33

Other potential sperm issues 34

Sperm Agglutination- Clumping of sperm 34

Varicoceles 34

Damaged sperm ducts 35

Testicular Failure 35

Chapter 6 Optimising Your Chances of Becoming Pregnant Naturally 36

Are fertility monitors and ovulation predictor kits useful? 36

How to time sex most accurately 38

What is the best sexual position for guaranteeing a pregnancy? 39

Douches, vaginal sprays and scented tampons 39

Antibiotics and yeast infections 39

Get in the best health of your life 39

Dairy? Junk Food? 40

Caffeine, nicotine alcohol and drugs 40

Is Alternative Health Useful? Acupuncture and Herbs 40

DHEA supplements 41

Other things to try 41

How to choose the sex of your baby 42

Chapter 7 We have tried for six months but it isn't happening: What tests do I ACTUALLY need (as opposed to the ones they tell me I need)? 43

When to see your doctor and what to expect 43

Female fertility tests and common issues 44

Standard Pelvic Exam 44

Waking temperature charting 44

Blood tests 44

HSG (Hysterosalpingogram) 45

Ultrasound 45

Endometrial Biopsy 45

Surgical options 45

- Laparoscopy 46
- Hysteroscopy 46
- Falloscopy 46
- Resolving Infertility 47
- Drug Therapy 47
- Surgery 47
- Four common female fertility problems 48
  - Make sure you are in control 49

Chapter 8 Assisted Reproduction: Decoded 50
- What procedures yield the best success rates? 52
- What actually happens in IVF, GIFT and ZIFT? 52
- Risk factors during IVF 53
  - IVF Success Rates 53
  - Stress and IVF 54
  - Other factors that affect outcome of IVF 54
  - Summary 54
  - First Test Tube Baby and the Future 55

Chapter 9 Yay! Early signs of pregnancy. OMG! What now? 56
- How much value do Pregnancy tests offer? 56
- C section vs. natural birth 57
  - Indications for C–section 57
  - Risks for the mother 58
  - Risks for the child 58
  - Recovery 58

Chapter 10 Dealing with miscarriages 60
- What can cause miscarriage? 60
  - Infections 60
  - Hormonal problems 60
  - Uterine abnormalities 61
  - Antibodies 61
  - How to know if you are having a miscarriage 61
  - Can I do anything to prevent the risk of miscarriage? 61
  - How soon can we try again? 62

Chapter 11: What if it all goes right? 63

Useful Websites 65

References 65

Introduction

There are few things in life as rewarding as starting a family and raising a child. The feeling you get when your baby smiles, when your baby takes their first few steps and starts to utter their first words cannot be described. Words like amazing, humbling, and exhilarating do not even come close. Only other parents know this truly indescribable feeling. For many it is such a life changing experience that life splits into two halves: Pre parent days and post parent days.

The purpose of this book is to help those of you who may be struggling to become pregnant for whatever reason. There is a whole load of information you will need to know before you go down the road of painful tests, expensive procedures and quite frankly many of them are unnecessary if you know and understand your body. There are many couples who are told they are infertile when in fact they are not. This book will help you identify everything you can do to maximise your chances of becoming pregnant naturally. If you do require medical help, this book will also take you through the logical steps of what tests you may need and when. It will discuss the rapidly changing world of assisted reproductive technologies to give you the knowledge to be able to work with the doctors to achieve a successful pregnancy quickly.

For the happy couple having a child together takes your relationship to another level. You have created something magical between you that is yours for life to nurture, teach and treasure. You will have started on an unfathomable journey that will teach you things about yourself that you were not expecting, it will challenge your patience and self-control beyond your limits and may teach you to live on very little sleep for a while!

Deciding to start a family is a big decision and as the cliché goes, it will change your life forever. Many couples are fortunate and conceive fairly quickly when they plan to.

However for many, the whole process is fraught with high emotions, disappointment, stress, anger and resentment. This applies to BOTH ends of the spectrum, whether you are:

- a young person who has "accidently" become pregnant without meaning to: having to face choices of telling parents and teachers, leaving school, abortion, adoption, not going to university and the on-going relationship(or not) with the father of the baby or
- a couple who weren't even trying, not ready emotionally or financially and became pregnant, accidently now facing similar decisions as above or
- a happy couple having decided to bring a child into the world then finding out these things do not always work to their timetable or finding out that one of you is infertile or finding out both of you are fertile with no problems, but it just is not happening for some unfathomable reason!

There are high emotions every step of the way. If you look at the statistics, very few babies are born at the "right" time. Most people never feel "ready" for a child. It never seems like the "ideal" time. Often couples say they could do with getting a bit more cash together, or just getting that promotion or having more time but most of us just adapt when it happens and muddle along somehow.

I presume by reading this book you may be either:

- looking to become pregnant soon and doing some research or
- you have tried already for a year or more and been unsuccessful and want to optimise your chances of conceiving naturally
- or maybe you have started down the road of medical assistance and want more education on the process, the options available and you want to know whether you are doing the right thing or not?

Wherever you are on your journey, this book will provide you:

- The latest information on reproductive health - we know so much more than we did 20 years ago - much more than your 5th grade teacher taught you
- How to massively enhance your likelihood of getting pregnant naturally
- Three signs to look for every month to time sex to perfection (More accurate than ovulation predictor kits!)
- Four things men can do to improve their fertility
- The five things you can do to increase your chances of success if you are seeking medical help
- Demystify the high tech methods of medical assistance (IUI, IVF) available and know what is right for you and when it is appropriate to consider medical options
- Increase your knowledge of the whole world of fertility and pregnancy so you can take control of the process rather than feel like you are on a treadmill of irrelevant and unnecessary tests
- How to cope with miscarriage and when it is safe to start trying again
- How to deal with the psychology of trying to fall pregnant and keeping your relationship together

Getting pregnant is based on a bit of luck, a bit of education, healthy internal bodily mechanisms (both the man and the woman) and many other uncontrollable factors. Maybe you are in the situation of seeking medical help and are being shunted from clinic to clinic, from waiting room to waiting room, being poked and prodded and tested for all sorts of conditions that you can't spell and that you never knew existed.

You may be in a state of confusion and helplessness with a slight bit of growing resentment every time one of your friends announces they are pregnant. This book will aim to cover all your options, explain the procedures and put the control firmly back in your court. Sometimes it is hard to get the right information out of your well-meaning doctors. You need to have as much knowledge as you can.

I know this because I have been through this process myself. It is so ironic isn't it? I have been through the years of ensuring I would not become pregnant, being "responsible", the years of career building and the endless search for "the one", coming close a few times and having a few near misses. I was a successful mid wife and had helped thousands of happy women give birth.

Finally I settled down with my gorgeous husband, we decided to go for it and take the plunge to become pregnant, expecting it would happen in one or two months. As the rest of my life had gone pretty well on schedule- why wouldn't this?

Suddenly I found it did not happen immediately. Oh well, I did not worry, maybe it will take three or four months? Maybe I am stressed? Maybe I need to eat more spinach? Maybe I need to stand on my head once a day? Maybe I should try acupuncture? All sorts of old wives tales and myths come to the forefront- I have tried them all!

To my absolute horror, it still didn't happen and eventually I relented and found myself at the mercy of the medical professions feeling completely like I should not be there. After all there was nothing "wrong with me". However before we knew it, my husband and I were on the treadmill of clinic appointments, unnecessary tests knowing there was nothing "wrong" but it just was not happening. All the tests came back perfectly clear with no problems. There must be another way. I did months of research in the libraries, bookstores and internet. There is a lot of information out there but it is difficult to assemble in the one place. Forums and chat rooms are full of well-meaning people but every case is different and even though it is helpful to know other people are going through what you are going through, they can only speak from their own experience.

Anyway through a significant amount of research, I learnt so much about my own reproductive system, the signals to look for which indicate your most fertile time, emotional consequences of infertility and the medical procedures on offer and when they are relevant to you. So that if you do need to seek medical help you can make informed decisions about the possibilities and be certain you are in the right place at the right time.

Personally I found it very difficult to get to the bottom of what help, if any, I really needed. I was often being pushed down a path which I did not really need or understand. Obviously there are large sums of money involved in many cases so it pays to do your research and not have unnecessary (and painful) tests you do not need. Please note I am not a doctor. Every case is different and there may be very valid reasons for you to seek medical help and take advice based on your condition. I am sharing what happened to me, the knowledge I gained so you can be more informed, optimise your fertility naturally but also work with your medical team if you need to in order to get pregnant fast.

This book will guide you through a logical pathway starting from:

- Before you start trying to be pregnant
- How to take control of your own reproductive health
- What to do if it doesn't happen
- What medical interventions are available and when they are appropriate for you

This book is NOT an encyclopaedia about IVF. IVF is simply one of the many treatments available and there are many more less invasive and expensive treatments available before you get to that stage.

This book is NOT an encyclopaedia of myths and legends of getting pregnant handed down by spinster aunts and nuns who knew no better.

I will try to make this book as informative and logical as possible, but keep it light and relevant. Education is the key, and if you pay attention you will know more about your body than most people and certainly more than what they taught you in school.

Many people are told they are infertile when they are not.

With a few minor lifestyle changes, many couples can become pregnant without tests and expensive procedures. The more you know and can control about your own body, the better chance you have of becoming pregnant naturally and avoiding the nasty procedures that lie in wait for the uneducated.

By the way 50% of infertility problems relate to the man and his sperm issues. Often it is the woman who is subjected to a myriad of painful, expensive and unnecessary tests only later finding out his little "swimmers" just ain't swimming! I include a chapter later on discussing male fertility problems and what can be done about them. So whilst I suspect most of the readers will be women, hopefully there is a willingness on your partner's part to get involved and do what needs to be done. If possible ask your partner to read this book too. It is important he has an understanding of the process and what he can do to help his natural fertility and support you when required. Hopefully you will both find this book concise, clear and very helpful.

I had a friend called Amy who was 33 years old. She and her husband had been trying for 14 months to become pregnant without success. She sought medical advice and found herself very quickly paying thousands of dollars for tests and procedures and eventually ended up on IVF. She went through 3 cycles before deciding to have a break. She needed to both financially and emotionally.

She sought my advice and after teaching her the techniques I will teach you in the next few chapters, she understood more about her own reproductive health, improved her husband's nutrition, they both cut out toxins, alcohol and smoking, she paid attention to her body's signals detecting her most fertile days and within 4 months she conceived naturally.

Even if you think you have tried "everything" and are currently undergoing some of the medical procedures available, still start reading this book at the beginning and try again to do everything you can naturally to be as fertile as you can.

Many books on becoming pregnant do not include the fertility treatments available. I have chosen to include both information on conceiving naturally and the medical options available. You both need to understand your bodies and what you can both do to optimise your chances of becoming pregnant naturally but also understand (if this fails) what your next option is, then your next one and so on.

Also some of the statistics thrown about there on the internet and by well meaning "friends" are simply outdated and wrong! For example a commonly mentioned statistic is that women over 35 years old have a 66% chance of getting pregnant in the first year. This comes from a study of birth records from 17th century France! This is totally irrelevant given our improved nutrition, understanding and general health, I will provide you with the updated statistics later in the book!

You will also need to be aware of possible psychological battles and irrational feelings you may have with yourself, with your husband/ partner or with your doctors so be prepared for these. You may find a support network helpful or maybe you have a friend or sister who has been through a similar experience. It can be so confusing and feel "unfair" when you have managed to control and excel at everything in life so far, you now want to plan and control pregnancy, birth and your child. This process may not fall into your schedule as easily as you would like. Remember to do your research but also keep a healthy dose of flexibility, humour and patience as this will be one journey you will never forget.

By the way, even though I was subjected to loads of tests, procedures and even two failed IUI's (intra uterine inseminations), I eventually become pregnant naturally at 38 years old and now have two healthy, happy and very noisy little boys and a lovely daughter who simply light up my life and for whom I am very grateful. I will explain throughout the book what happened to me and how I came to be pregnant when at one point it was not looking promising.

I hope you enjoy the book, get the results you need and please tweet me your success stories.

Jessica Randolph

@pregnancybible1

Chapter 1 What To Do Before You Start Trying

Anxiety about pregnancy can begin before you even start trying to get pregnant. In fact, for women, the anxiety can start as a young girl, looking at pregnant women's tummies wondering how on earth a baby comes out of there and knowing that one day that might be you! As you find out more about how the whole process works through your teenage years, panic can set in especially when we see horrific scenes on TV from labour wards and hear horror stories from our well-meaning older sisters, cousins, friends and whispered conversations.

Sometimes it may seem that ignorance was bliss. In our grandparent's and parent's day, people seemed to just throw away birth control methods (if any) and got on with it. I am sure not many knew anything about the murky world of ovulation, basal temperatures or sperm count- let alone the intricacies of sperm motility! However while it is tempting to look back on the past with rose tinted glasses, all was not bliss and many couples did remain childless for a variety of reasons. Today many of these people would certainly be able to have children, some of them naturally with a just a little education and some with a little medical assistance.

Things are different in today's modern world. Both men and women tend to marry later. We all have more opportunities and choice about travel, careers, and who we wish to settle down with. In fact some might say we have too much choice which in itself might be a problem as we delay starting the process to be absolutely sure we have found "the one" and that we are actually "ready". Some of you will have found "the one" a little later than you thought, some might have been focused on getting a solid foundation in their career first and some maybe just were not in a position either financially or relationship wise to even consider starting a family.

But whatever the reason, when you decide to start a family, education is the name of the game because without this your efforts may be random and you may find yourself at the mercy of the medical system unnecessarily. This book will show you how to take control of your own reproductive health. Many so called "infertile couples" are not infertile at all. The two biggest reasons for not conceiving naturally (besides medical problems) are the two reasons which are easiest to address:

- Mistiming sex by a just day or so
- Poor vitamin and mineral intake

There are a whole host of other reasons which could also be interfering with your chances of becoming pregnant. This section will help you address all the things you should be doing prior to conception to maximise your chances of success.

Six Months Before Conception

The health of the parents is critical to becoming pregnant and having a normal healthy baby. Did you know the brain and nervous system of an embryo start developing incredibly early, around two weeks after conception? It is not good enough to wait until you become pregnant before you start looking after yourself. You do not find out you are pregnant until three-four weeks after conception or even longer in many cases. By then, your unborn child may already have a birth defect. The embryos heart and brain are already developing and are very sensitive to the effects of alcohol, smoking, drugs and other toxins that could cause major problems.

The earlier you start to plan for pregnancy, the better health your baby will have. For example Folate, one of the B vitamins drastically reduces the risk of neural tube defects. It is most effective taken before conception. In fact to NOT take this routinely if you are thinking of starting a family is foolish. Just 0.8 mg a day before pregnancy and during the first 6 weeks of pregnancy can dramatically reduce your change of baby neural tube defect, brain and spinal cord defects and spina bifida.

Incidentally **both** the man and the woman should take a good multivitamin regularly three-six months prior to conception. The health and strength of the sperm is equally important in becoming pregnant and giving the unborn child a strong start with all its nutrients in place.

This is not being obsessive, it is just plain smart and responsible!!

Will The Odd Cigarette Cause Any Harm?

Smoking and drugs need to be completely eliminated. Smoking sharply increases incidence of infertility. It will take at least three months after you stop smoking to get back to normal. So please stop now; no sneaky ones either! Most people know that pregnant women should not smoke but it is important prior to conception in **both** the man and the woman to quit smoking. The sperm and the egg are both affected by smoking and result in low birth weight babies. There is also a strong link with asthma in children.

Surely Caffeine Is OK? I Need My Coffee To Function!

Caffeine also adversely affects fertility. In men caffeine has a more severe effect on fertility. Five or more cups of coffee or tea per day reduces fertility by half! Both men and women should limit caffeine to one cup per day. Combined bad habits like someone who is a heavy drinker, heavy smoker and heavy caffeine user may become effectively infertile. Some studies show that with these bad habits it can take an amazing seven times longer to get pregnant than a healthy couple.

What About Alcohol?

A glass or two of beer or wine a couple of times a week is fine but certainly going out on a massive drinking binge is not advised. In fact over three drinks a day increases the risk of infertility by 60%. This is MASSIVE! Also men's heavy drinking is even worse for fertility than women's! Both of you need to lighten up immediately on the booze if you are trying to get pregnant.

Does Sleep Affect Fertility?

Sleep is extremely important. Sleep deprivation kills everything from your mood to your immune system. Get at least eight hours daily and even go for ten hours on weekends if possible. Also vitamin D from natural sunlight boosts the immune system and boosts fertility. Sunlight also helps you sleep better.

All these factors are important for your health and the health of the embryo. Nature is quite cunning in that if it feels you are drinking heavily, on drugs and smoking like a chimney and neglecting your diet, it will make it a little harder to become pregnant. I know there are plenty of examples of cases where drug addicts and heavy smokers become pregnant but there are always exceptions to the rules. There are also many cases of "infertile" couples who decide to give up these toxins after months of trying to conceive and failing then three months later, they do fall pregnant. In general the message is to optimise your health before you conceive to make becoming pregnant as easy as possible and ensure the best possible health for the embryo.

Best of all, these things are easy and cheap to implement and in fact will save you money if you stop smoking and reduce drinking.

Coming Off Birth Control

If you have been on the Pill, you will need to come off a couple of cycles before you start trying to conceive. This is important to make sure you are ovulating normally again and to allow your uterine lining to build back up (hormonal birth control methods can thin it out). Birth control injections like Depo-Provera can take up to nine months to leave the body and you might have irregular cycles during that time. If you have an IUD (inter-uterine device) you should be able to conceive shortly after having that removed. If you use condoms or chart your cycle for birth control, you simply time unprotected sex on a "fertile day" and you can potentially conceive immediately.

Are Environmental Hazards Relevant To Me?

Some women worry about the radiation from their computer affecting them especially if they have a job where they sit in front of the screen all day. There is no evidence that a computer screen affects your reproductive health. Though men should not use a laptop balanced on their lap due to both the heat and potential radiation right next to their exposed sensitive bits.

Do a quick check of your kitchen cabinets. Plastics can leach into food and deliver unwanted doses of chemicals. Bisphenol-A(BPA) a chemical found in soft plastics mimics oestrogen. A study has found that women who have high level of (BPA) in their body have more unusable eggs during IVF. Chemicals are more likely to leach out of heated plastic so if you cook leftover rice, soup or leftovers in your microwave, use a glass or ceramic container. Buy a stainless steel water bottle and drink most beverages out of a glass rather than a plastic bottle.

How Much Exercise Is Healthy When I Am Trying For A Baby?

Moderate exercise every day is key to maintaining a healthy body. Exercise helps to burn off excess body fat and also helps in normalising your hormone levels. Exercise will also decrease stress levels and help give you the ability to cope with everything life throws at you. Evidence has shown that vigorous exercise five or more hours a week enhances fertility. Women are 40% less likely to have problems with this regime. Vigorous exercise does NOT mean walking around the block or doing zumba once a week. It means activities like regular jogging, running, cycling >10 mph, strenuous dancing, hard swimming, hard weights sessions- something where you sweat and your breathing rate increases. In addition, some yoga positions have been found to be very beneficial to improve the fertility health of both women and men.

But while moderate exercise enhances a women's fertility, being an exercise fanatic can impede it. Studies have shown that an excessive amount of exercise resulting in low body weight and low fat levels may give you in irregular periods, irregular ovulation and luteal phase deficiencies (I will discuss luteal phase in detail later).

Attention runners: A surprising cause of a short luteal phase is running. If you are a runner, you may want to cut down the mileage before trying to get pregnant. A short luteal phase will affect the length of your cycle and may contribute to miscarriage as the embryo needs enough time to implant in the uterus.

How Important Is Body Weight?

Being overweight or underweight can both affect the chances of ovulating normally in a woman. In order to ovulate, women need at least 20% body fat. Being underweight can prevent ovulation altogether. Olympic runners, gymnasts and many professional ballet dancers lose their periods altogether and then often have difficulty conceiving later. Women who are underweight may want to consider putting on some weight if they find that menstruation tends to be sporadic. Additionally, being underweight may indicate that you will have a hard time producing the extra amount of energy required for pregnancy. Maintaining a healthy weight before conception is therefore advisable.

Being overweight though is not the answer. This can alter your cycle by causing excessive production of oestrogen. Overweight women with ovulation and menstrual cycle problems may want to lose some weight if they are having troubles conceiving. However, overweight women do not necessarily need to lose a significant amount of weight in order to help their conception rates. Even slightly reducing your weight can dramatically increase your chances of conceiving. An Australian study found that, as soon as a group of obese women lost almost 20 pounds, their bodies began to spontaneously ovulate again.

What Foods Are Most Important In My Pre Conception Diet?

Eating a healthy, balanced diet is essential when you are trying to conceive. Even if you need to lose some weight, do not starve yourself, depriving your body of nutrients. Instead drop the highly refined, processed foods and reach for fresh fruits and vegetables, rich in anti-oxidants and minerals and lean meats.

Both vitamins C and E play key roles in female and male fertility. A high intake of these vitamins may increase sperm count and increase sperm motility in men; while in women these vitamins can reduce stress on the eggs and the reproductive organs. Sperm need to be able to swim efficiently in order to reach the egg. Foods that contain antioxidants, vitamin E and selenium will help improve the sperm motility and make them better swimmers. Some research shows that if you are trying to conceive, it is wise to avoid sea food as the high level of mercury may be responsible for abnormal semen and decreased fertility.

Many infertility issues crop up due to hormonal imbalances. This can be avoided by removing all processed flours and sugars such as white bread, pasta, pop, candy, and sugary juices from the diet.

Eating foods with a low glycaemic index such as fruits, vegetables, and beans; lean protein like yoghurt, chicken, tofu, and turkey; and essential fat including walnuts, sesame seeds, and extra virgin oil at every meal helps maintain the hormonal balance in the body and improves the functioning of the reproductive organs.

Certain herbicides and pesticides sprayed on crops have been found to have drastic effects on fertility. In particular, xenoestrogens, a type of oestrogen, found in environmental chemicals and pesticides may disturb the hormonal balance in women and lead to infertility. Choosing organic foods whenever possible will help you to avoid this chemical as well as others.

In addition, visit your doctor and make sure all your childhood jabs and inoculations are up to date.

While much of this advice seems like common sense, you would be amazed at how many people do not do it. Even if you have to make some changes gradually, do start today. I can count hundreds of couples that I have dealt with personally who have been told they were infertile who made dietary and lifestyle changes who then became pregnant naturally within 3-6 months. It is worth it and it will definitely help your quest to have a lovely, healthy baby.

For me, I thought it would be easy. But when I tried to cut down on coffee, biscuits and chocolate, I did stumble a bit at first. I kept drinking coffee throughout the day thinking "one more cup won't hurt". It really did require some serious will power and reminding of my goal (to have a baby) to break these habits but I am sure it did help me become pregnant a few months later.

Chapter 2: Back To School: Important Lessons In Reproductive Health (this will contain at least five things you did not know!)

Despite the panic we all had as young people when we first started dating about how easy it was to become pregnant, women are actually only fertile for a few days each month (It was probably a good thing that we didn't know this information then!).

This is one of the reasons it is such a shock for couples trying to have a baby when it doesn't happen straight away. Many couples do take several months of "trying" before the joyous event occurs.

Is infertility increasing?

Most people know someone who has conceived using IVF or is trying IVF. It is unclear whether infertility is increasing or whether people are simply seeking treatment in higher numbers. It is probably a combination of increased awareness of medical help available, couples delaying starting the process and fewer stigmas attached to seeking help when required.

The standard medical definition of infertility is "not becoming pregnant after one year of unprotected intercourse". However many of these couples are NOT actually infertile. Some may just need to time sex more accurately or change their lifestyle a little.

For example my friend Molly, was trying to become pregnant for over two years. She was told she was infertile and was advised to start IVF treatment. The doctor had told her and her partner to have intercourse around day 14 as that is when the woman ovulates. After over a year of trying this she still was not pregnant. However once I explained to her how to chart her cycle properly and understand her own body, she found she did not ovulate until day 20. The "day 14 intercourse" routine was a complete waste of time. It was not achieving their objective which was conception. Armed with more accurate information Molly became pregnant after two months of accurately timing sex around ovulation (rather than an arbitrary day 14)!

The point is and I am sure you have grasped it, is that well-meaning doctors are taught that women ovulate at day 14. However in reality, while majority of women might ovulate day 14, that does not help you at all if you ovulate on a different day! You could be completely fertile, you could just be timing intercourse wrong resulting in a wild goose chase of expensive procedures, tests and IVF for no reason at all. During this book I will teach you how to chart your cycle so you will be able to pinpoint when you ovulate and how you will know when you are most fertile.

Remember doctors are trained to look for disease. If you do not fit into their "norms" it is assumed you have a disease and the process of endless tests will begin. The truth may be very different. You may be perfectly healthy but simply have an irregular cycle or a longer luteal phase.

The Technical Bit: The Four Primary Reproductive Hormones

Hormones often have a bad reputation! They are often blamed for angry, irrational behaviour which is a little unfair. They control most of the internal systems we have and are extremely important. Hormones are biochemical substances that are produced in one area of your body and carried in your bloodstream to send signals that trigger responses in another part of your body. Here is an overview of how they work together during the menstrual cycle. This is extremely important as it will help you pinpoint when ovulation occurs. Also some of the treatments some of you will be on will be hormone based treatments.

Every menstrual cycle is under the influence of FSH (follicle stimulating hormone) and about 15-20 eggs start to mature in the ovary. Each egg is encased in its own follicle. The follicles produce oestrogen, the hormone responsible for ovulation to occur. A race progresses for one follicle to become the biggest. Eventually ovulation occurs when the dominant ovary releases an egg. The other eggs that began to ripen disintegrate. It is fairly arbitrary which ovary releases an egg. It was previously thought that they took turns but this has been shown not to be true. Although it averages about two weeks, the race to release an egg can take anywhere from about eight days to a month or longer to complete. The primary factor that determines how long it will take to ovulate is how soon your body reaches an oestrogen threshold. The high levels of oestrogen will trigger an abrupt surge of Lutenising Hormone (LH). It is this LH which causes the egg to burst through the ovarian wall.

After ovulation the egg tumbles out into the pelvic cavity and is swept along the fallopian tubes. Following the release of the egg, the follicle collapses becoming a yellow body or corpus luteum. This corpus luteum remains behind and starts producing progesterone. The corpus luteum has a finite life span of twelve-sixteen days. It is a problem if the corpus luteum lifespan is less than eleven days and is one reason for infertility which I will discuss later.

Progesterone (another hormone) is incredibly important for a woman's fertility because it does three things:

1) Prevents the release of all other eggs
2) Causes the uterine lining to thicken and sustain itself until corpus luteum disintegrates twelve-sixteen days later
3) Causes the three primary fertility signs to change- waking temperature, cervical fluid and cervical position.

Cleverly the progesterone prevents multiple pregnancies by preventing the release of more eggs every day. Sometimes one more egg does escape and if it is fertilised, it results in fraternal twins (non identical twins born from different eggs).

The first part of the cycle from menstruation to ovulation is called the follicular phase. Its length can vary considerably. The second phase from ovulation to the last day before new period starts is the luteal phase. It usually has a finite span of twelve-sixteen days.

What Happens At Conception?

Assuming fertilisation does not occur, the egg remains alive for 24 hours then dies. If fertilisation does occur, it usually happens in the outer third of the fallopian tube (not in the uterus as popularly believed) within a few hours of ovulation. The sperm may have taken several hours to get there. About a week later after fertilisation, the egg reaches the uterus and burrows into the lining.

In order for conception to occur three things must be present: an egg, a sperm and a medium in which the sperm can travel. This medium is the cervical fluid which acts as a living conduit to direct the sperm through the cervix. Women produce cervical fluid under the increasing levels of oestrogen in the first part of the cycle. Because sperm can live for up to five days, it is possible to have intercourse on Monday night and become pregnant on Friday night. As soon as the fertilised egg starts burrowing into the uterine lining, it starts releasing a pregnancy hormone called HCG (human chorionic gonadotrophin) which sends a message back to the corpus luteum to remain alive beyond its sixteen days, continuing to release progesterone to sustain the nourishing of the lining. After several months the placenta takes over, not only maintaining the endometrium, but providing all the oxygen and nutrients the foetus needs to thrive. It is the HCG hormone that pregnancy tests are looking for in the urine to signal a positive pregnancy.

One of the reasons for false negative pregnancy tests is the test is done too soon before the egg has implanted or before the HCG has had time to rise enough to be detected in the urine or blood stream.

The Three Primary Fertility Signs (Get to know these well and you may save yourself thousands of dollars in unnecessary tests).

Most women are painfully oblivious to what happens to them each and every cycle, when they are actually fertile or not and the actual process of conception. Most of us do not pay attention in school during reproductive class as the whole thing is just too embarrassing for words and has most of us, including the teacher squirming and wanting the whole thing to be over and done with as quickly as possible. In many cases, the teacher simply does not know much either!

Fertility treatment can run into tens of thousands of dollars and have serious emotional costs that need to be factored in. It is important before you go down this route that you have tried everything you can naturally to become pregnant. As I have mentioned before there are many couples who are sent down this route unnecessarily through lack of knowledge on their part.

In my experience, I was fairly quickly ushered into IUI (Intrauterine insemination) without any discussion of my diet, lifestyle or natural fertility signs. IUI is a fantastic procedure for many people and will result in successful pregnancies. I am simply highlighting that many of you may not need it if you improve your general health. Also the likelihood of it working will be greater if your general health is the best it can be.

Remember even though most medical professionals do their best, for some of them, it is a business and they can be rather quick to initiate treatments. Remember also most doctors simply go on the fourteen day ovulation cycle and if you do not fit into this "average" most of their advice will not apply to you. You must know your own body and your own signs. This is so important- and by the way- not difficult.

So here are the three fertility indicators that will provide you with important information.

1) Waking Basal Body Temperature

Basal body temperature tends to be the lowest temperature your body experiences throughout the day. Women tend to have lower temperatures during their follicular phase (pre ovulation) under the influence of oestrogen, then higher temperatures in their luteal phase under the presence of progesterone released by the corpus luteum after ovulation. If pregnancy does not occur, the disintegration of the corpus luteum causes a fall in basal body temperatures and another cycle begins. If pregnancy does occur, the corpus luteum continues to function for the first trimester and the temperatures remain high. After the first trimester the corpus luteum is no longer required and is replaced by the placenta and temperatures return to their pre-ovulatory level.

The first thing you need is a basal body temperature thermometer. Do not use a fever thermometer- it is just not as sensitive as it needs to be for our purposes. Make sure you have one that reads $1/10^{th}$ of a degree. You will need to take your temperature first thing when you wake up. Do not get up and go to the toilet first. Place it at your beside table to make sure you remember and write it down straight away. Your body temperature changes over the course of a day (see table 1.1) and varies with different activity levels.

Table 1.1 Normal Body Temperature Changes Over An Average Day.

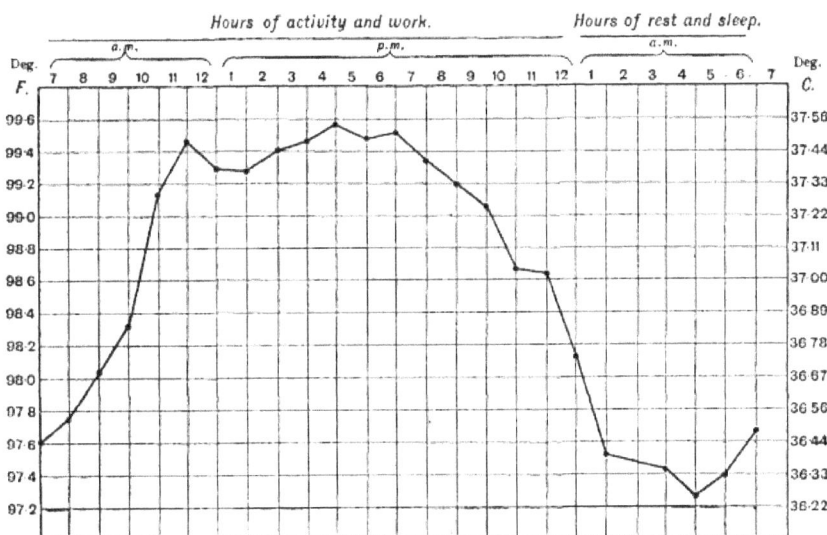

If you have regular menstrual cycles, it will be assumed that you ovulate normally but in some cases, women can have regular cycles and NOT be ovulating at all or be irregular. Recording basal body temperatures will determine if you are ovulating normally and will determine the length of your luteal phase.

One of the most common mistakes is trying to get pregnant by timing intercourse by these basal waking temperatures. A woman's pre-ovulatory waking temperature typically ranges from 97-97.5 F with post ovulatory temperatures rising to 97.6-98.6 F(36.1-37C) See Table 1.2. After ovulation the temperature will stay elevated until your next period twelve to sixteen days later.

Temperatures typically rise within a day or so of ovulation and are the result of progesterone which is a heat inducing hormone. So by definition higher temperature indicates that ovulation HAS ALREADY occurred. The last day of lower temperatures is the day of ovulation. Temperature will rise the day after that and stay high until the first day of your period (or will continue to stay high if you are pregnant).

Table 1.2 Basal Body Temperature over a month (Celsius)

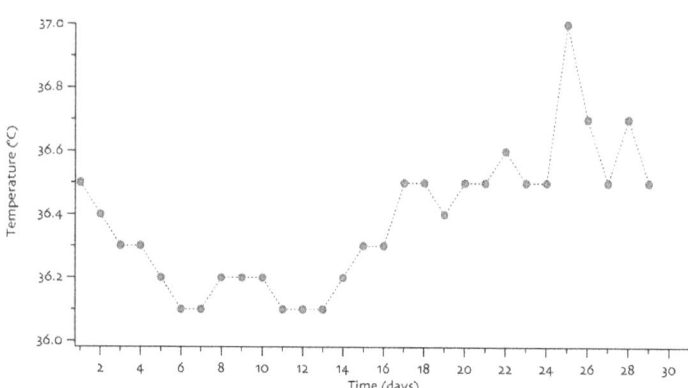

When you look at the chart, stand back and observe the overall pattern. Do not worry too much about day to day fluctuations. Also be warned: other factors can cause increased temperatures too like: drinking alcohol the night before, having a fever, getting less than three consecutive hours sleep the night before or electric blankets.

Stress, medication, strenuous exercise or travelling can make your cycles longer. Note: these factors can only affect the first phase(follicular phase) of your cycle not the second(luteal phase) which is constant.

What does this mean?

This means that basal temperature is NOT a good indicator of when you ovulate but it confirms that it HAS occurred. This is important to know. But this tool is useless at letting you know when to time intercourse because the change in temperature occurs AFTER ovulation, when it is too late.

Basal temperature recording will determine how long your luteal phase is- whether you have at least ten days from ovulation to menstruation which is necessary for implantation to occur. This knowledge could prevent a painful and unnecessary diagnostic test such as endometrial biopsy.

Recording your basal temperature will also let you know if you are pregnant when you notice 18 days in a row of high temperatures. Women are often misled to think they are not getting pregnant when in fact they are getting pregnant but they are miscarrying in the next week. Sometimes it is hard to tell as a miscarriage can be mistaken for a normal period but if you charted your temperatures you would know that the bleeding is a miscarriage.

This is vital information to give your doctor if discussing your treatment. For example, if you were starting from scratch you may be forced down the route of infertility treatments until the doctors realised that getting pregnant was not the issue but holding onto the embryo was the problem. This is usually due to a short luteal phase which is treatable. This information gained from a cheap little thermometer could save you thousands of dollars on unnecessary fertility treatments and lots of heart ache. With the right treatment you could be pregnant and carry to full term.

Why should I chart my temperature after I am pregnant?

Continuing to chart your temperature after you have a confirmed pregnancy is important. If you notice a sudden drop in temperature (after 18 days of high temperatures) it is a very strong indicator that you could be miscarrying.

Charting will also allow you to determine your accurate date of conception rather than medical estimates. This will determine your actual due date more accurately. This is important because many women are unnecessarily induced at labour or have mistimed amniocentesis because the doctor got the timing wrong- again usually based on averages of 28 day cycle with day 14 ovulation.

2) Critical Factor in Fertility Success: Cervical Fluid

Cervical fluid is a critical success factor in fertility. Cervical fluid in a woman acts like semen in a man, to help transport the sperm up into the cervix. Without this, the sperm are literally useless and die very quickly. Cervical fluid is present only during the woman's fertile phase which only lasts one to three days. It provides an alkaline medium to protect the sperm from the acidic vagina. It is worth noting here this fluid is different to normal sexual lubrications.

There is an observable pattern of change in cervical fluid in all ovulating women. Once you learn to observe these subtle differences you can identify very easily when your most fertile time is. When a woman is extremely fertile, her cervical fluid (some call it mucus) becomes very wet. Some of you will find this topic a bit squeamish or unpleasant but you better get used to it because when you do become pregnant you will be close up and personal with a whole load more of your lovely child's smelly, stinky bodily fluids at highly inconvenient times!

As your cycle progresses your cervical fluid changes in texture and volume. These changes occur because of the influence of the hormones mentioned above. The best time to observe your cervical mucus is when you go to the bathroom. You should be able to see it when you wipe yourself with toilet paper. You need to observe the consistency and colour. Right after your period, you may observe nothing near the vaginal opening. It may be fairly dry or produce just a bit of moisture. This is not your fertile time. A few days later you may develop a type of cervical fluid described as "sticky". The critical point it is that it is not wet. This is not your fertile time either. The next type a few days later is "creamy" or lotion like and it is cool to the touch. This is not your fertile time either. The next type is so wet and watery you have difficulty handling it. You are almost there now. The final and most fertile fluid resembles raw egg white. It is extremely slippery and it can stretch from 1-10 inches. It feels like lubricant and in some cases it may even be red tinged which is called ovulatory bleeding. This is your fertile time and you know what you and your partner need to be doing! In fact you need to continue to have intercourse daily or every second day until you do see a definite shift in basal temperature which confirms ovulation has occurred.

Finally in the day or so before menstruation women may notice a wet, watery sensation. This is due to a drop in progesterone that precedes disintegration of lining of the uterus. The first part of the endometrium to flow out is typically water hence the watery sensation.

So begin checking every day after your period has ended. Start writing down what the quality of the fluid is: dry? creamy? sticky or slippery? Some women also notice their vaginal sensations throughout the month. This can also be an important indicator of fertility- you may feel slippery fluid, dry or sticky.

Women in their twenties may have four-five days of this fertile fluid, women in their thirties maybe have a day or two.

Make sure you can differentiate between actual cervical fluid and basic vaginal secretions. A little trick is the glass of water test. Normal secretions will simply dissolve in a glass of water whereas cervical fluid will form a blob that sinks to the bottom (Hint: do this in private!).

What if there is no cervical mucus?

That's ok- you might have to touch inside the vagina to find it which is fine. Also do not obsess about how many days you have it. You only need one day to get pregnant but you do need to carefully observe the signs and act quickly when you get the signal.

If you actually do not produce much cervical mucus you may wish to try a lubricant (some medications like Clomid dry up your natural cervical fluid). Do not use just any lubricant. Most of them actually kill sperm on impact. Lubricants like ProXeed actually mimic egg white and do not kill sperm.

3) Cervical position (optional)

The cervix also goes through changes during a cycle. Many of you can attest to the fact that intercourse can be painful one time but lovely the next time when you try it in exactly the same position. Why is this? The cervix prepares for pregnancy every cycle as well. It acts as a biological gate through which sperm can pass on their way to finding the egg. It becomes soft and open during ovulation. But outside of ovulation it is firm, low and closed. You can palpate your cervix if you want to. Many women do not wish to do this. I would only recommend it for those women whose temperatures do not fluctuate enough to give them a solid clue about their fertility. It is best to have two indicators. For instance: Basal temperature and cervical fluid or cervical fluid and cervical position.

Pick two of these three signs to monitor and chart daily to accurately know when you ovulate and when your most fertile time occurs.

Here is an example of a cervical fluid chart.

Phase & Stage	Sensation	Cervical Fluid look
Pre-ovulatory	Dry-Light Moisture - INFERTILE	No observable mucus.
Fertile	Moist or sticky	White or cream in color, thick to a little stretchy. Breaks easily when pull.
Highly Fertile	Slippery, wet, lubricated	Thin, watery, transparent, like egg white. Increase in total.
Post-ovulatory	Dry, Moist or Sticky - INFERTILE	Thick, opaque white or cream-colored, very less in amount.

To make it more accurate write down what happens each day and the day number. So you should have 28-40 entries each month. Start to look for patterns and see how it relates to your temperatures as well. The chart will let you know when your most fertile day is. Generally this is the last day you produce fertile cervical fluid (stretchy egg white fluid).

Your most fertile day occurs a day before or the day of ovulation itself. Remember this will be the one or two days **before** your temperature shifts. You may have already noticed that you will only be able to determine your most fertile day AFTER the shift in temperature. Also it is a day or two BEFORE your cervical fluid and vaginal sensation have already begun drying up. Also be aware your most fertile day is not necessarily the day of greatest **quantity** of cervical fluid. Always look for **quality** of fluid- it MUST be stretchy raw egg white material.

Secondary fertility signs

There are also secondary fertility signs which you can observe. These are perhaps less reliable but some of you may notice repeatable patterns. If you do, please chart them to give you more clues. These signs occur around ovulation:

- Mid cycle spotting
- Pain in the ovaries
- Increased sexual feelings
- Swollen vulva
- Water retention
- Increased energy level
- Breast tenderness

What a hassle!

Some of you I know are already screaming at the book- "what a hassle!" and "I can't be doing that every day!!" However it will take less than a minute a day and may be all it takes to avoid six months of painful procedures or thousands of dollars spent on potentially unnecessary infertility treatment.

Instead try to think of charting as a privilege which gives you so much control over your body, gives you more information than the medical profession will give you and will also guide you to having appropriate tests if required at the right time.

Charting your cycle will also give you control over gynaecological procedures if you need them because you will be able to spot abnormalities easily. For example knowing if you have an infection, spotting, what is normal and what needs medical attention.

But What If I Have Irregular Cycles?

As you know not everyone has a regular 28 day cycle! Also a cycle may change from month to month within an individual. Cycles may also vary throughout your life depending on whether you are breastfeeding, coming off the Pill, adolescent or approaching menopause. It also varies if you are stressed, travelling, heavily exercising or ill. The beauty about charting your cycles is that you will know exactly when you are fertile or not ovulating. You are in control.

Once you begin to chart you will notice patterns, even if they differ from the norm, they may be more obvious to you. The point is if you chart and write down your temperatures and notice your cervical fluid, you will know when you are most fertile which a whole lot is better than random attempts at becoming pregnant, failing miserably and feeling like something is wrong.

Chapter 3 Age and Fertility. Phew! Not As Scary As I Thought

You have probably heard the frightening statistics about dramatically diminishing fertility beyond the age of 35 years for women. Did you know this comes from a study from 17th century France? Remember at this time in history, most people died by the age of 50, they had poor diets and minimal reproductive knowledge or medical assistance. This is completely irrelevant to us today.

It is easy to become panicked and stressed about the whole ageing thing and the pressure to be "getting on with it". But try not to let statistics scare you. In another example a recent newspaper article stated "only 2% of babies are born to mothers aged 40 and over".

This makes it sound like women of 40 years only have a 2% chance of having a baby! This is wildly wrong. This statistic only comes about because most 40 year old women are trying desperately NOT to have any more children rather than women who CANNOT have children after the age of 40. They have either had their families or do not want children.

So please banish this from your mind and let us examine the more recent data. A 1990's study found 50% of 30-39 year old women were pregnant naturally after 3 months, 82% became pregnant within a year and at end of 2 years 90% were pregnant. A U.S. study, released in June, 2013 appears to back up the argument, suggesting that 80% of 38 and 39-year-olds get pregnant naturally within six months of trying.

Another study released earlier this year, which tracked Danish women having sex during their fertile periods, reported similar figures: 78% of 35 to 40-year-olds got pregnant within a year. It followed 2004 research that suggested of those having sex twice a week, 82 per cent of 35 to 39-year-olds conceived within a year - just 4 per cent fewer than those aged 27 to 34.

Of course there is plenty of scientific evidence that a woman's highest fertility is in her twenties but do not despair if you are older and do not be scared by statistics from three centuries ago. Simply you will need to get educated, chart your signals, get you and your partner healthy and be outcome focused. You may not have the luxury of ten more years of random intercourse if you want to create a little "mini –me". Be sensible, know what is going on, time sex accurately and go get it.

In our favour also is better health, testing kits, improved reproductive knowledge and education. The most recent evidence points to the fact that women in their late 30s and early 40s can conceive naturally. It may take 3-6 months instead of an instant result. If you are over 40 years old, your best chance is to try to become pregnant naturally as IVF does favour younger women. It is imperative that BOTH of you take prenatal vitamins, have a good diet, quit smoking, remove toxins, get enough sleep and reduce alcohol.

There is also a lot of data coming out of IVF clinics as they have plenty of patients to compile data on. They found that

- 50% of women who undergo IVF aged 30-35 years go home with a baby;
- 30% of women aged 35-39 years go home with a baby;
- 14% of women aged over 40 years go home with a baby.

Please note: these results are for one cycle attempt only so with multiple cycles, the results will be better. If you are over 40 years the medical advice is try naturally for three months then seek help as you do need to get on with it. In the initial stages there will be a lot of tests to go through and you may find that there is a small problem that can be easily fixed.

The reality is that miscarriages are more common in women over 40 years. The statistics are 10% incidence for women under 30 years old, 18% for women aged 35-39 years and 34% for women aged 40-44 years.

The man's age is also crucial and the integrity of the sperm does diminish in men over 35 years. You are more likely to have a Down's syndrome child and suffer miscarriages if the man is over 35 years. There is not much you can do about this except be as healthy as you can, eat well, get enough sleep and take prenatal vitamins. There are scans you can take when you are pregnant to test for any birth abnormalities.

Another statistic you may have heard is there is a higher risk of birth defects when the women is over 35 years old. This is blown out of all proportion-there are risks but the risks are minimal. The statistics prove in women over 35 years old, 99.5% of babies are born normal and healthy; in women aged over 40 years old 98.5% of babies are born normal and healthy.

So yes, fertility is better in younger women but as long as you do some preparation with respect of your health, arrange correct timing for intercourse, you have a very good chance of conceiving naturally after 35 years old.

Why women are delaying pregnancy until their 30s

Anyone who asks this question should be shot! I mean do they think it is a deliberate attempt to make life more difficult for ourselves? Do we plan to be in a doctor's surgery listening to a lecture on "fertility is better in your twenties"... Yes, we all know that! Yes, ideally we will all be pregnant in our teens or our twenties...or even earlier if you really want to talk about ideal age of fertility which is probably around 15 years old.

However can you imagine a school or university student, with no money or career, who has not settled down yet with a suitable partner, not quite knowing how to stand on their own two feet bringing up three kids? It is just not very responsible nor very possible for many of us.

Some of us are childless at 35 years and older either because we want to be, or because we haven't found "the one" yet or we thought we had found "the one" only he turned out not to be, so we had to begin the whole darn process again.

However to keep a healthy balance of truth, fertility does start to decline at age 27- but not by much. After 35 years and especially after 40 years the decline does become steeper. We do need to be mindful of this but there are many happy stories of women giving birth in their forties-remember we are generally better educated, better nourished and in better health than previous generations. So our chances are much higher.

Both men and women at some point have to face the reality that you will not be fertile forever, consider how many children you want, how spaced you would like them to be and work with probabilities. Remember if you plan on breastfeeding you probably won't be at top fertility again until you wean the baby. This is why many babies are spaced two years apart.

The psychology of trying to get pregnant

It can be a complete roller coaster of emotions trying to get pregnant, waiting weeks to see if it worked, testing with pregnancy kits, charting daily, being unsuccessful, picking yourself up and starting over from scratch next month. It can take over your body, mind and soul and consume every waking thought. It is easy to say "just relax" but even though general worrying and stress will not make you infertile, it will make you crazy!

Throughout the "trying to get pregnant" process, couples will often go through extreme emotions of excitement, anticipation, disappointment, anger, frustration and worry. Sometimes it causes immense strain on a relationship and sometimes the pent up feelings can be turned on the other person. Be careful that your frustration and anger at not conceiving do not get turned on your partner in a "blame game" or that your whole lovemaking experience becomes clinical and routine.

When you and your partner first started to try for a baby- it was probably more along the lines of let's stop contraception and in a month or two we will be pregnant. What happens when your conversation becomes "how long before we consider adoption? What if one of you wants to try surrogacy?" Even the strongest relationships can be put under immense strain by continual disappointments, anxiety, depression or blame.

Focus on what attracted you to each other in the first place, try to keep open communication channels, respect that people deal with their emotions differently to you- if you are still struggling, talk to a counsellor who might be able to give you independent view and get things back into perspective. Many relationships do break up due to infertility so be aware of this and respect it. Do not wait until it is too late to save it.

Obviously you need to develop ways to cope and make things easier on you. Take as much action as you can to make you feel in control of the process. Read books, get educated, buy kits, take supplements, do the testing, do the charting and of course the best bit-have sex. After you have ovulated and done all you can that month, focus on relaxation. There is literally nothing you can do now until your next cycle. Do not spend every minute worrying. It will not help.

Keeping a journal is a great way to deal with your emotions. Definitely talk to a friend or support group but keeping a journal that no one else will read is a powerful way of dealing with emotions that are too scary that you may not want to discuss with anyone else. Anxiety caused by psychological trauma can result in "physical and biological dysfunction."

The main problem is women think and contemplate far more than men. It is our nature to worry more and to stress more. This is why women are twice as prone to depression as men. After ovulation there is nothing left to do, so make sure you exercise, see friends, show gratitude, get sunlight every day, take omega 3 (at least 1000mgs), get enough sleep at least 8 hours (preferably 10 hours), mediate, breathe and laugh.

It is ironic that throughout most of your life, you probably do not think much about babies or even notice them when you are out. However when you are trying to have one, you will see new-borns and toddlers everywhere; you will notice that pregnant women seem to be following you, simply to torture you. Many of your friends will be announcing their pregnancies with such joy. Sometimes this can be extremely painful to be around. Obviously be happy for them but do not deliberately put yourself in situations you know you will find painful like baby showers and christenings. And then there is the unfairness of unwanted teenage pregnancies that will simply drive you crazy!

Nurture your relationship with your partner

At first trying to have a baby brings you closer together: great excitement thinking about future possibilities, thinking of fantastic names, imagining your child's first day at school and of course an excuse to have more sex. But once the initial excitement dies off to be faced with month after month of disappointment you may start to feel increased pain and worry but he seems to be fine. Does he not want a baby too? Does he not care about me? Is he really "the one"?

Many books write "don't expect him to "get it"". He probably won't. Because pregnancy does not happen inside men, they are more removed from the whole process. Also they are programmed to be stoic and not show emotion. Of course some of them will be more demonstrative and will show their caring side, but some of you will just have to accept- they just aren't that into it as you.

He should, of course, listen to your concerns, provide emotional support, understand that you may be slightly neurotic or hormonal from time to time and be involved as much as possible in getting the result you both want. This will require sensitive communication from you to explain exactly what you need from him- as most men don't "get it", it does not happen to them and they for the most part can only focus on one thing at a time.

If they are watching the football or out with their buddies, they are not thinking about the baby. Don't worry, do not freak out. Also remember if they see you freaking out, they actually do not know what to do, so mostly they will either do nothing, pretend they do not see you or walk away to allow you "space" to get yourself together. The problem is most of us just need a hug right then. So you may view him walking off or ignoring the problem as uncaring, cruel and selfish and as a result, get even more worked up and angry! Then the problems escalate and both sides feel misunderstood and isolated.

Sometimes there is literally nothing the male partner can do except support the woman. Ladies remember it is difficult for your partner to see you very upset all the time, maybe in pain, injecting yourself daily with hormones, going through constant disappointments if it does not work month after month. Both parties need to be supported and understood.

Make sure you still make time for each other away from the pressure of trying to get pregnant. Do not make this your one topic of conversation, continue your hobbies, keep it light and see other friends. Make time together now as you know there will be much less time together when you do have the baby.

Remember to make love, not just have sex

As you know by now the women is only fertile for a couple of days a month so you do need to work with military precision and be precise, disciplined and accurate about this but the rest of the month please chill out, make sex fun, take the pressure off and just be yourselves. Stay positive, know you are doing everything you can to be as healthy as you can, surround yourself with family, great friends, fun trips away, whatever you can do to ensure you are not bogged down in a spiral of monthly disappointments that eventually eats you up and destroys you.

When couples do experience relationship breakdown over infertility, it is usually because they have lost the emotion of lovemaking. Sex has become a function, a chore, a process and even a painful reminder of failure rather than a source of pleasure and closeness.

Keep talking to each other, and give each other some slack. You are both going through a difficult time and it will be natural to snap occasionally. Just resolve it as quickly as you can and get back to a place of close communication, support and continue your journey together.

Make the effort to keep your romance alive. Continue to have nights out, notice the efforts the other person has made, complement each other, give hugs, bring flowers home or leave little notes for the other person to find. Always appreciate the other person. It is stressful for both of you.

Chapter 4 Will Anything I Do Adversely Affect My Fertility?

We have discussed age, being as healthy as you can to aid conception and being aware of your own body and the signals it gives you regarding your most fertile days of the month. But is there anything which you do on a day to day basis which works against you?

Is there anything you could change in your lifestyle to accelerate your quest for a successful pregnancy?

Will Excessive Stress Affect My Fertility?

Stress does not adversely affect your fertility but it may delay ovulation.

Sure everyone will tell you "just relax, it will happen" which is highly irritating. The only thing you should focus on to become pregnant quickly is accurately predicting ovulation then making sure you and your partner act quickly.

This is being intelligent- using the scientific evidence and the knowledge we have to hand. Being too laid back, waiting for it to "just happen" may just not work.

A certain amount of stress is normal especially with modern couples and the stresses of working, seeing friends, family, paying bills, commuting, your boss and relationships in general!

It is commonly quoted that stress leads to infertility. Also the reverse is true, infertility leads to stress! Simply leading a busy life leaves a couple little time or energy to have intercourse frequently enough to increase their chances of conception. Remember it does not actually have to be frequent sex but simply well timed sex.

Another way stress affects fertility is how it affects when ovulation occurs. Stress dramatically affects the functioning of the hypothalamus, the gland which is responsible for so much of the reproductive system. It is also responsible for appetite, temperature and emotions. It regulates the pituitary gland which controls the reproductive hormones FSH and LH. Schedule time for yourself to regularly de-stress and keeps things in perspective- perhaps yoga, meditation, a walk along the beach or deep breathing.

I know for me, I am a bit of a control freak. I do everything at high intensity. I work, hard, I exercise hard and I party hard. While trying to get pregnant I gave up partying hard to focus on getting rest and looking after myself better. But I noticed actually I still did not give myself any down time. I eventually forced myself to do one meditation class a week and one yoga class a week. I had always seen these pastimes as a waste of time and felt I should be in the gym or running. But I was surprised at how doing them regularly gave me such a sense of control and relaxation. During the class I had time to visualise everything being alright and working out in the end.

I can't say for sure whether these classes were responsible for me being pregnant naturally but I am sure they really helped. They gave me a deep sense of peace that I was really grateful for. I highly recommend them to anyone trying to conceive.

Will Depression Affect My Fertility?

Depression however DOES adversely affect fertility. It has a big negative impact. Depressed women are half as likely to get pregnant as those who are not. You may feel down from time to time but how do you know if you are depressed? If you are sad and crying all the time for more than two weeks; that's depression. Try to change your scene, go on holiday or try relaxation techniques rather than medication in the first instance. If it continues you may need to talk to a doctor or a counsellor.

If you work long hours in a stressful environment and don't sleep enough, this will have negative effects on trying to get pregnant. Try to relax before bed, certainly no working or watching television in bed. Try to relax with your partner, read a fiction novel, have a hot bath and chill out at least an hour before bed. Good sleep and enough sleep is imperative to ensure that you conceive.

Why are some women more fertile than others?

There are some women you just want to punch in the face when you are desperately trying to conceive. Like those who helpfully say "he just has to look at me and I get pregnant" or "Silly me, I get pregnant on every method of birth control."

It appears that some women just are very fertile. This could be due to having shorter cycles so they ovulate more frequently allowing more opportunities, or those with an extremely long luteal phase or those with extremely fertile cervical fluid. I'm afraid it is "just one of those things" in life that is unfair. Even if you have looked after yourself all your life, eaten well, exercised, not smoked or taken drugs, it may or may not take a long time. This cannot be predicted.

There is also some element of the "chemistry" between your eggs and your partner's sperm. This is not scientifically proven just anecdotal evidence probably due to lack of participants in the study.

However there are some women who just cannot get pregnant for years of trying with their partner. Both have been through tests and there is no known cause of infertility. Later on they break up for some reason. She meets someone new, and falls pregnant immediately.

(By the way I am not saying this is an alternative! Just an interesting quirk of life!)

Chapter 5 Male Fertility

You now understand why charting the three signs for optimum female fertility is so important for pregnancy achievement. Now we need to delve into the world of male fertility, potential problems and how to resolve them.

Over half of fertility problems are caused by sperm issues! In many cases girls, it is NOT your fault! Sperm tests are quick, cheap and inexpensive. So if you have tried diligently for 3 months around ovulation to become pregnant have a semen analysis done as soon as possible. Be careful to insist on a proper sperm analysis. It is not just sperm *count* which is important but *motility and form*.

This means it should also tell you what percentage of those sperm are normal shape and size (morphology) and what percentage are rapidly moving forward (motility). An analysis of these three factors will tell you whether your partners count is normal, low or infertile. Sperm count is considered normal if when the magic moment occurs his ejaculate contains 20 million sperm per millimetre and if the total sperm present is approx. 150 million in half teaspoon of semen.

Sources and labs vary so much about what is considered normal morphology and motility. You will have to discuss this with your doctor. If the man's sperm count is sub fertile, it makes sense to repeat the tests a few more times in the following weeks as an occasional low sperm count can occur sometimes in a man with generally normal sperm due to illness, fatigue or stress.

Help! We have a sperm issue- What can be done?

Initially make sure your partner is following the general rules for good testicular and sperm health. He should:

- Wear boxer shorts with lots of air circulating rather than tight lycra pants
- Supplement his diet with multivitamins containing magnesium, selenium and vitamin C. This dramatically assists the strength of the sperm motility
- Avoid hot tubs, saunas and hot baths as sperm are very sensitive to heat
- Avoid too much time on a bicycle which also diminish sperm count due to the constant bumping and bruising of the testes and heat generated around the scrotum.
- Avoid certain situations like standing in front of a pizza oven or a fire for 8 hours

Remember it may take three months after making changes for a new generation of healthy sperm to mature. So if your partner has added prenatal vitamins to his diet or stopped smoking and you are not pregnant in a month- you must keep going. Do not give up. It takes time for the body to eliminate toxins and the good nutrients to build up to an effective level.

- If the man's sperm count is normal: Have intercourse every day that you have wet cervical fluid and wet vaginal sensation through to and including the day of your first rise in temperature. Of course the closer you time it to your most fertile day (last day of wetness), the more likely you are to conceive.

- If the man's sperm count is low: Have intercourse every other day that you have egg white fluid or wet vaginal sensation through to and including the day of first rise in temperature.

The reason you should have intercourse less frequently is to allow the man's sperm count to build up again to higher levels. In fact you should abstain from intercourse until your cervical fluid is slippery, enabling the sperm count to reach normal levels prior to ovulation.

All men whether they have normal or marginal sperm quality should abstain from any type of ejaculation at least a few days before your most fertile days to maximise the chances of the most sperm with the strongest swimmers entering the uterus at the right time.

Finally most sperm is in the first part of the ejaculate. Men should try to penetrate deeply to deposit sperm as close as possible to the cervix. It is a long way for the little fellas, I am sure they appreciate any help they can get!

Supplements for low sperm count

Zinc deficiency is a common contributor to low sperm count so encourage your partner to add this to his diet and add daily supplements. Zinc is contained in seafood-especially oysters, beef, lamb, spinach, cashew nuts, pumpkin seeds and chicken. Also a deficiency in vitamin B, selenium, magnesium is highly linked to poor sperm performance so supplement these too. Arginine –an amino acid has been shown to be very helpful for markedly improving sperm count and motility. Try 4 g a day of powdered arginine.

Hormonal treatments

There are also hormonal treatments available for men with low sperm count. Men also can have hormone deficiency due to inadequate or erratic release of FSH and LH (the same reproductive hormones that we discussed earlier for women). It is sometimes possible to treat with gonadotrophins but male hormonal problems are very complex and often difficult to treat.

Hi Tech treatments

There are also high tech ways of introducing the sperm to the egg if these treatments fail. Sperm can be removed directly from the man's epididymis using an ultra-thin needle. It can then be inserted directly into the egg (which has been removed from the woman). This process is called intracytoplasmic sperm injection (ICSI). Fertilisation is achieved in a petri dish then the embryo is transferred back into the uterus.

TESA (testicular sperm aspiration) is a procedure involving a needle biopsy of the testicle in which a sample of tissue is taken directly from the testis and used to extract sperm for IVF or ICSI.

PESA (Percutaneous sperm aspiration) is a procedure involving a needle into the epidiymis in an effort to locate and aspirate a pocket of sperm.

Other potential sperm issues

Sperm Agglutination- Clumping of sperm

This is a common condition post vasectomy reversal. Sometimes the operating surgeon will claim to have performed a "successful" reversal as there are sperm present in the semen however due to post-operative inflammation, antibodies become present resulting in the sperm clumping together, rendering them effectively useless.

Steroids are sometimes prescribed to suppress the immune system. In some cases adrenal hormones may restore fertility.

There has been an incredible recent study with men who have been diagnosed with clumping sperm post vasectomy reversal. In the control group who made no changes, there were no pregnancies. In the test group the men took supplements of calcium, magnesium, manganese and 1000mg vitamin C they all got their partner's pregnant within 5 months.

Caveat: The study only contained a small group of people but fascinating nevertheless and if taking some supplements for a few months negates the need to go down the IUI or IVF route it is certainly worth trying!

IUI (intrauterine insemination) is the most common treatment for sperm clumping. It involves sperm washing which tries to separate the best swimmers. The sperm is then placed in the woman's uterus via a catheter allowing the egg and sperm to meet hopefully in the fallopian tubes or the uterus. This means the sperm do not have to swim so far so increases the chances of conception.

If IUI is unsuccessful, the couple may wish to try IVF or GIFT (which I will discuss later).

My husband and I tried IUI and had two failed attempts. He had marginal sperm count and I had no known problem. This does not mean IUI is not a good method to try and it certainly should be tried before IVF as long as the woman's fallopian tubes are open. I know of a handful of friends who have undergone IUI with a successful result and have happy, healthy babies without going through IVF.

It is worth noting though that the success rate for IUI is 15%. This quite low but as you can imagine there are all sorts of reasons for this statistic. One of the reasons is the quality of the actual sperm, the quality of the egg, the health and age of the parents. The IUI cannot change that, it just tries to bring the sperm and egg closer together. Another reason is the timing must be very accurate. The same timings apply to IUI as to timing intercourse. You cannot wait until ovulation as the egg will have already left the ovary and it will be too late. You need to time it a day or two before ovulation as the sperm can survive for up to 5 days so it is there to meet the egg when it leaves the ovary. Charting will allow you to pinpoint the exact day that you should undergo IUI. Also there are ovulation predictor tests which can also aid you as to the right day.

Varicoceles

Varicoceles are an abnormal enlargement of the venous plexus in the scrotum. These are due to defective valves in the veins that drain blood away. The symptoms include aching pain in the scrotum, feeling of heaviness in the testicle, shrinking of the testicle, visible enlarged veins.

30-40% of all infertile men have these which cause venous blood pooling in the scrotal sac. Surgery will help 80% of men with this problem.

Damaged sperm ducts

Blocked sperm ducts account for 15% of male infertility. Often this is caused by a sexually transmitted disease. Most of these cases require surgery to eliminate the blockage or scarring.

Testicular Failure

This is fairly common. The reproductive hormones released from the pituitary gland are normal but the testes do not respond and therefore do not produce sperm. This can be caused by illnesses like mumps, STD's surgery, tumours, sports injury and drug use. There does not seem to be any effective treatment that will improve sperm production where there are none. However if there are some sperm present, fertility drugs can improve their numbers. Also there are high tech procedures that can retrieve sperm direct from the testes even if the man's sperm count is zero.

A diagnosis of male infertility can be one of the hardest challenges a man can face. For some, it can be devastating. Not being able to father a child can make a man feel like he's failing at one of his most primal responsibilities. They can feel emasculated, guilty and sick when they hear their mates are becoming fathers. It is difficult to talk about with their friends and the usual response from their mates is something unhelpful like "let me know if you need any help with the wife" which is sometimes unbearable.

There are more support groups around for men these days but if your partner is suffering psychologically try to encourage him to talk to a counsellor or find a support group.

Chapter 6 Optimising Your Chances of Becoming Pregnant Naturally

At school most of us got the impression we could become pregnant from kissing boys, or holding hands. Life is so ironic! Most people spend years in their twenties trying to avoid becoming pregnant with a few hilarious stories to tell along the way: the condom breaking during the peak moment of intercourse, a diaphragm flying across the room as you attempted to insert it, a few sleepless nights wondering if you were pregnant when an unexpected passionate clinch had you doing the deed without precautions. Yet ironically, by the time you actually want to become pregnant, you may find it is not so easy after all! Then you find out the egg can only live for 12 hours a month!

Anyway, this is the reality like it or not! So before you race off to the doctor and enter the world of infertility treatments you need to make sure you have optimised your chances of becoming pregnant naturally.

Here is a summary:

- Know when you ovulate. And you need to know this in advance. (Remember charting temperatures ONLY tell us when we HAVE already ovulated- by then it is too late). You need to know this precisely, or you could be thinking you are infertile when you are simply missing your fertile day by a few hours. It can occur anywhere from day 7 to day 40.

    If you have regular cycles you may want to try the "sex every other day between day 7-21 method". But if this is not practical, you need to carefully predict the two most fertile days which are 2 days before ovulation. To do this you need to choose a method which is accurate and easy for you to follow. I have discussed at length charting and looking for your body's own fertility signs- temperatures, cervical fluid and cervical position.

- One of the most important factors in getting the sperm successfully to the egg is quality of cervical fluid. If you need help with this, you can use ProXeed which has the same acidity as cervical fluid. Do not use traditional lubricants as these actually kill sperm. A recent study found in men with low sperm count who used ProXeed, 21% of their wives became pregnant with ProXeed compared to 2 % without. Incidentally, undergoing IUI also bypasses the cervix and the need for high quality cervical mucus.

- Out of interest the other possibility some couples use is actual egg white. I am serious. It is exactly the right medium with the right amount of protein you are looking for. Try it if you are game!

Are fertility monitors and ovulation predictor kits useful?

These are a useful to aid our charting. Of course some women use them *instead of* charting their own body's signs. In my experience, knowing your own body and charting the signs gives you the most accurate information regarding your fertility and day of ovulation but the kits do act as a helpful back up and sometimes as confirmation. These kits are not gospel. They can sometimes be slightly off the timing and can be misleading. By implementing the information from earlier you already YOU will be much more accurate and save yourself money. However they do have a place and some women find them very helpful.

Ovulation predictor kits detect the LH (luteinising hormone) surge which your body secretes approximately 32 hours before you ovulate, although it may be 12-48 hours before hand (which is why you should measure and chart your temperature as well). These kits are cheap from the drugstore or chemist. You should start testing around day 10. However if you have long cycles (29-42 days) you may ovulate between day 15-28. The kits only come with 7 sticks- you will need to buy more.

Another caution is some women with short luteal phases may be testing much earlier than when they actually ovulate which may lead her to think she is not ovulating when actually she has simply miss-timed it. Again if you chart your temperature, this will be no mystery.

However many of you will prefer to use these kits rather than do the charting and observe your bodily changes. If so then here are some factors to be aware of:

1) The kits test the LH surge (luteinising hormone) that precedes ovulation. They do not indicate whether the women **has definitely ovulated**. In some cases the woman may have LUFS (luteinised unruptured follicle syndrome) where they have the LH surge but the egg actually never pops put.
2) A woman may have false LH surges in which she has mini peaks of LH before the real one causing her to miss-time intercourse too early. The sperm needs to survive long enough for the release of the egg. In addition if the woman has PCOS (polycystic ovarian syndrome) her body may continually produce false LH signals.
3) The kit does not indicate whether the woman has suitable quality cervical fluid to allow sperm the correct medium to move toward the egg. In addition by the time the kit does show a surge, the cervical fluid could be starting to dry up.
4) The kits are only as accurate as the person using them. They may also produce false signals if they are damaged due to heat, transport or storage.
5) Some fertility drugs interfere with the accuracy of the tests.
6) Women over 40 years can have elevated levels of LH. A testing kit should only show a surge of one day. If you see an LH surge of more than one day, the test is invalid.

Fertility monitors cost more. They cost approximately $150-200 which some say are more accurate and you also have to buy the sticks at approximately $35-$50. Here are some examples of two of them:

1) Clear plan easy fertility monitor (£120 - $190)

This is an electronic system that works with a standard urine test to monitor your cycle. It analyses both LH and oestrogen within the urine to tell you which phase of the cycle you are in. If used correctly it can effectively predict ovulation about 1-2 days before it occurs.

2) Cue II Saliva Monitor (£210 - $327)

This device measures electrolytes in your saliva. Use daily from day 1 until it signals you are within 7 days of ovulation. You begin having sex every other day while using a small vaginal sensor which confirms that ovulation has occurred.

3) A newcomer to this world is the OV watch which detects levels of chloride in your sweat. Chloride levels dip about four days before ovulation then rise again. The OV watch can give you more warning about impending ovulation than ovulation predictor kits.

There are plenty of others on the market ranging from $500-$1000. Whilst some of these may be helpful, the most important thing is the discipline to be consistent and get to know your own body. I believe the most accurate is the self-monitoring I have discussed in earlier chapters but some women do find that they do prefer the testing kits for extra confirmation.

It would be great if getting pregnant were as easy as making it happen when you felt the time is right. Yet for many people it requires more knowledge than we were taught growing up. Remember a lot of people today are told they are infertile when in fact they and their doctors have simply misunderstood their cycles. For many couples- just timing it right results in pregnancy. For many couples just upping their vitamin intake and reducing alcohol and smoking results in a successful pregnancy. For many a little knowledge, discipline and understanding massively reduces immense cost and insane amounts of unnecessary stress. I know I have stated this already but it is so important it is worth repeating.

How to time sex most accurately

When to have sex is the most crucial thing for getting pregnant. If you do it daily, you may skip this section! But if you are a "once a week" couple, you might be missing the fertile couple of days each and every month. Even if you do it twice a week (you are still probably the envy of your friends) but you are still likely to miss the two most fertile days every month.

You do not need to have sex constantly and excessively until you are both burned out- you can get pregnant from once a month sex but it has to be timed correctly. Many couples who try for many months without success are just simply timing it wrong.

Having sex the day you ovulate is just too late. You MUST time it a day or two beforehand. Remember the short life span of the egg is just twelve hours. It is possible to miss it completely. If you or your husband are away for a night with work, then have sex the next evening it could be way too late! Even if you discover you ovulated in the morning then have sex that night, again, you could be too late. Also studies found pregnancies conceived the day of ovulation lead to a higher chance of miscarriage.

As I discussed earlier, you do not know you ovulated until after you've ovulated. The only way to make sure is to have sex every other day when you see egg white mucus. Keep going until your temperature rises.

Reproductive sex can be a beautiful thing. Make sure it does not become a chore or mechanical and boring. There are no worries about a condom breaking, there is an amazing sense of purpose and hopefully you have found "the one" and are deliriously happy. Keep it fun, some couples find the stress of doing it on demand with constant disappointments every month too difficult. If this happens, take a few months off trying by the calendar and relax for a while. Then come back refreshed and relaxed.

What is the best sexual position for guaranteeing a pregnancy?

More studies are required and there is not much evidence to support any sexual position one way or the other. The current thought is traditional missionary position is best as the man can get himself closest to the cervix. It may be worthwhile for you to lay there for half hour afterwards to allow his sperm to travel up before you get up and start rushing around. However there are also studies that show that if his sperm are strong swimmers, they will already be on their way even if the woman gets up straight away and goes jogging!

In this instance, my advice is to do what feels best, remember to keep it fun and varied. The most important factor to worry about and track is exactly the right day and time to have intercourse.

You don't need to stand on your head for half an hour after making love in order to get pregnant. If you are timing intercourse at the right time, the sperm will swim up the cervical fluid rapidly no matter what position you are in.

Douches, vaginal sprays and scented tampons

These alter the natural acidity of the vagina such that sperm can't survive. Do not use these.

Antibiotics and yeast infections

Antibiotics often kill the good bacteria along with the bad leading to overgrowth of candida which is a type of yeast that renders vaginal environment inhospitable to sperm. Counteract this with eating yoghurt containing acidophilus or ingesting acidophilus tablets.

Get in the best health of your life

I have mentioned diet earlier in chapter 1 but I will return to it here briefly because it is so important. Actually do this and sort your diet out. Do not just pay lip service and many of you will become pregnant without doing anything else. When trying to get pregnant your body should be as healthy as possible-this is essential for both you and your partner. Limit refined foods, excess sugar, caffeine and products with additives. All of these can impede your livers ability to metabolise hormones. Eat a well-balanced diet of wholesome foods which can eliminate many problems. In addition heavy milk consumption may adversely affect fertility and should be reduced.

Yes I hear some of you screaming …"but there are overweight teenage girls out there who get pregnant by living on a diet of Coca-Cola, cocaine and tobacco- that's not fair!"

Yes there are exceptions to every rule but there are many more couples who struggled to become pregnant, then changed their diet significantly and within 3 months, the job was done and they were planning baby names!

The research on weight is clear: Women who weigh too much and women who weight too little will take longer to get pregnant- twice as long for overweight women and four times as long for underweight women. Maximum fertility is best at BMI (body mass index) 20-24.

Starts taking prenatal vitamins three months before trying to become pregnant so adequate nutrients build up-especially folate, iron and B6. Do not wait until you are pregnant- it will be too late to prevent neural tube deficits. Also consider taking a fish oil supplement. There is evidence to suggest that those women who consume omega 3 have smarter babies. There are other reasons as well to include omega 3 in your daily routine. The benefits of omega 3 go way beyond brain development. People who take it have significantly less heart disease and less depression.

Pre pregnancy you must focus on healthy eating. Often in the first trimester all intentions of a good diet go out the window and you will crave starchy foods, sugars and fat. This pre pregnancy diet is so important many call it a 12 month pregnancy and I think they are right as a lot of preparation should begin at least three months beforehand.

A recent study found those who ate a diet of healthy natural foods with minimal chemicals and preservatives had **92% less chance of PCOS** (polycystic ovaries) than those who ate white bread pasta, sugary drinks and pizza.

Should I eat purely organic food? Yes if you can for your own general health as well, but there is no actual medical evidence of a link between organic food eating and improved fertility. However it does make logical sense.

Dairy? Junk Food?

Many books advise against dairy or at least seriously cutting down. Yoghurt is a better choice if it contains probiotics but avoid those with added sugar or sweeteners.

Two types of food increase risk of ovulatory infertility: sweetened fizzy drinks and trans fats. Studies show women with high levels of trans fats were 80-90% less likely to get pregnant from IVF. If you do not know what contains trans fats think: cookies, cakes, most junk food and margarines.

Caffeine, nicotine alcohol and drugs

If you have unexplained infertility you should both consider reducing or eliminating caffeine, drugs, alcohol and nicotine from your diet. They interfere with the ability to conceive and the man's sperm production.

Is Alternative Health Useful? Acupuncture and Herbs

Alternative medicine is extremely popular amongst women trying to get pregnant however studies have shown no difference in results with or without alternative medicine. There have been no studies on Chinese medicine and pregnancy. If you know anyone trying desperately to become pregnant you will know that they usually are willing to try anything - chiropractic, massage, naturopathy, yoga, reiki, meditation or chanting. There are so many that it is impossible to list them all.

Many women do try acupuncture treatments and there are many successful anecdotes. However there are no medical, scientifically validated studies.

This does not mean that it does not work.

It simply means there have been no conclusive studies into it. If you know someone who has tried alternative health and it has worked for them, apply a logic test- does it seem like it will work for you?

Also make sure there are no side effects of possible harm. If in doubt, avoid it but if there is no harm done and it makes you feel more relaxed and in control, be all means try it.

If you do have success with one of these, do tweet me and let me know.

DHEA supplements

Here is a story from a 42 yr. old woman who underwent IVF to store her eggs but only produced 3 eggs which is considered low. She started taking DHEA, an inexpensive hormone supplement. She started taking it without telling her doctors.

4 months after taking it, she produced 6 eggs and 6 months later she produced 14 eggs and 9 months later she produced 18 eggs.

Doctors started suggesting it to other women who did not produce enough eggs. One lady had several failed IVF cycles, then went to the doctor for nausea- he found she was pregnant naturally. There is evidence that there is improved pregnancy rates with DHEA and best of all, it has been shown to cut the miscarriage rate in half in women over 35 years.

There is no evidence of birth defects and women produce a higher amount of DHEA anyway during pregnancy as it is a naturally occurring hormone.

The recommended dose is 25 mg a day. It takes 4-5 months to work. Research is still in initial stages (the women in the original study took 75mg daily).

Other things to try

Avoid drugs that dry up cervical fluid like antihistamines, cough mixtures containing anti histamine, progesterone and Tamoxifen. If you must take Clomid, take oral oestrogen to compensate for its drying effects. But oestrogen should never be taken without fertility drugs because it may inhibit ovulation.

You could try taking expectorant cough syrup that which helps liquefy mucus in the lungs and also makes your cervical mucus wetter.

Take 5000=8000IU of vitamin A daily. Some women develop wetter more fertile fluid with such a regimen- but take medical advice as high dose vitamin A can have side effects.

How to choose the sex of your baby

I am sure most of you do not mind if you have a girl or a boy as all you want is a happy healthy baby.

But some parents have a secret desires for a boy or a girl or sometimes one of each. Dr Shettles sold 1.5 million copies of his book in 1970 on how to guarantee a boy or a girl. The book has been updated in 1996 and 2006 with co-author David Rorvik. The theory goes because boy (Y) sperm are lighter they swim faster and get to the egg first. Girl sperm (X) are slower but live longer. So sex further from ovulation should produce more girls. The book claimed an 80% success rate. However before you rush of and buy the book, it has been proven not to work. In fact more recent studies prove the opposite is true.

There is a 2008 study which found women who conceived boys ate more protein, folate and iron and 2250 calories a day. Of 133 specific foods studied, the largest difference was breakfast cereal! 59% had a boy. Also upping your quantity of potassium rich food helped swing the odds in favour of those wanting a boy: bananas, spinach, potatoes and oranges, milk cheese and yoghurt.

If you want a girl, the best results came from supplementing with calcium.

However only two techniques have a proven and reproducible 80% success rate in determining whether your baby is a boy or a girl:

1) Pre-implantation genetic diagnosis (PGD) and
2) Microsort

PGD is used with IVF. It extracts a cell or two from an embryo while still in the petri dish. The chromosomes are analysed and only the ones with the desired sex are implanted. Ethics are heavily involved. It is mostly used for family balancing, couples who have a family history of inherited genetic disease, carriers of gender linked genetic diseases or couples who already have a child with an incurable disease and need compatible cells from a second healthy child to cure the first.

Microsort is a similar process of sorting out the X and Y chromosomes and implanting only those of the desired sex.

Chapter 7 We have tried for six months but it isn't happening: What tests do I ACTUALLY need (as opposed to the ones they tell me I need)?

When to see your doctor and what to expect

The standard definition for infertility is actively trying for over a year but no pregnancy. However, I think the more realistic guide is if you have been trying for six months timing intercourse *accurately around ovulation* and nothing has happened, see your doctor. Many studies show it takes two-seven months to become pregnant even when everything was timed exactly right. However I will assume for this chapter that you do your charting, you do have intercourse at exactly the right time and you have tried for six months without success and have now decided to progress to the next stage which is involving a doctor or fertility expert and discussing the next steps.

There are many treatment options available through major technology breakthroughs and these are improving all the time. Sometimes there is the temptation to think that only through very expensive and invasive procedures like IVF can a couple become pregnant once they are over 30 years old but this is very untrue and sometimes counterproductive. Modern methods requiring artificial ovarian stimulation and high dose hormones can sometimes impede or delay the pregnancy they are trying to aid (through drying out cervical mucus or poor timing of procedures).

Remember seeking help or getting some tests done does NOT mean one or both of you is infertile. It does not mean at this stage that you need IVF treatment. It is important to get the initial tests done as these do take time and it may be that something is discovered that is very simple to address. It may be a case of antibiotics to clear up a low grade infection for one of you or an IUI procedure because his sperm are not swimming well. The majority of couples do NOT need IVF treatment even though it is much more readily available, talked about, with less stigma attached to it.

Make sure you are still charting, testing and doing all you can naturally with good diet, plenty of sleep, sunshine and positivity. Even if you decide to get medical help, keep doing all you can naturally as it is not uncommon for a natural pregnancy to occur once you have scheduled yourself in for an IUI or IVF treatment. Even though I have spoken about it at length, you will be surprised at how many do not chart! As well as identifying when the accurate time to have sex is, charting will also help you identify if there are any issues like anovulation (which means you do not ovulate), lack of cervical fluid, excessively short luteal phase and recurrent miscarriages. All are extremely valuable information.

Susan and Tim started trying for a baby at 37 yrs. old. After 3 months of trying they decided to see an infertility expert. They were impatient. Within 6 months they underwent IVF and had twins. 5 months after the birth she tried to work out why her period had not started back and found out she was pregnant again-naturally this time. Was IVF necessary the first time?

There are various factors which need to be present at the right time to become pregnant. If any of these are missing, pregnancy will not occur:

- A woman who is ovulating
- A man with sufficient sperm production (number, motility and shape)
- Intercourse with ejaculation
- Sperm transport and fertilisation
- Efficient embryo transport and successful implantation into the uterine wall

Female fertility tests and common issues

If you believe you have nothing wrong, your charting reveals nothing wrong, but you have not become successfully pregnant after 6 months then proceed to having your partner's semen analysis done. Remember 50% of fertility issues are a result of problems with sperm. Get this testing done first as it is quick, cheap, and painless and will identify half of the fertility problems immediately.

I have already discussed the tests for the man in a previous chapter so this chapter will mainly focus on the female tests.

Standard Pelvic Exam

Initially you will need a standard pelvic exam to check there is nothing wrong with the uterus, ovaries and cervix such as fibroids, cysts or infections. You will be asked your medical history.

If this is all clear then progress to diagnostic tests for endometriosis, uterine and fallopian tube abnormalities, cervical problems and dysfunctional cycles.

Waking temperature charting

As you know by now this will give you and your doctor information about whether:

- You are ovulating
- Your luteal phase is long enough i.e. longer than 10 days
- You have a thyroid problem
- You have become pregnant but are miscarrying- sudden drop in temperatures after 18 days of high temperatures

Blood tests

These will test whether your hormone levels are normal- FSH, LH, oestrogen and progesterone. You may be asked to have an AMH (anti-mullerian hormone) test. This is a test of ovarian reserve or "remaining egg supply" and estimates how many years fertility you have left. It is a simple blood test and will give you a number between 1-30 which is a rough indication of the number of antral follicles you have left in your ovaries. A fertility doctor can also do an ultrasound to tell how many antral follicles you have left.

An antral follicle count of 10 or less is considered "diminished reserve".

Does this mean that every woman over 30 years old should have this test?

No, because low ovarian reserve does not mean you can't get pregnant- it simply means the hyper stimulation required for IVF doesn't work very well. So even if you get the test and they tell you it is low- do NOT be distressed. It does mean IVF may not be as effective but many studies of women conceiving naturally find that ovarian reserve DOES NOT predict who gets pregnant and who does not. So if you are not requiring IVF, you should not require this test at this stage.

I heard of a lady called Nina through a friend of mine. She had an ovarian count of 8. She was 39 years old at the time. Obviously she was quite distressed at the low ovarian reserve as she and her husband had decided they wanted a family. A few months later she had an ultrasound which showed only 5 follicles left. She cried into her pillow for days, thinking that was the end and she would never have a baby.

However 1 year later she was worried she had hit the menopause as she did not get her period. She did a pregnancy test (just in case) and found she was pregnant. Over one year later, presumably having even less eggs left and aged 40 she became pregnant.

HSG (Hysterosalpingogram)

This tests whether you have any blockages in your fallopian tubes. This shoots dye through the cervix and uterus to see whether it spills out into the pelvic cavity. This uses X-ray technology to look for any damage or blockages in the uterus or fallopian tubes. It also looks for uterine fibroids, endometriosis and scar tissue.

This test can sometimes clear blockages in women with blockages in their tubes. The test takes 10 minutes; it can be painful so best to take pain killers beforehand and you may notice spotting or cramping afterwards. Most women will be advised to have this test as a routine.

Ultrasound

This is the only way to confirm ovulation has actually occurred. It is useful in detecting LUFS (Luteinised Unruptured Follicle Syndrome). This is discussed later.

Endometrial Biopsy

This determines whether the uterine lining is sufficiently developed during the luteal phase to be able to sustain a fertilised egg. This is usually performed a couple of days before the woman's period. A tiny piece of uterine lining is removed and examined. This test can be uncomfortable due to partially dilating the cervix.

Surgical options

If nothing abnormal is found there are surgical procedures you may be advised to try in order to pinpoint the reason for infertility.

Laparoscopy

This is primarily performed to identify endometriosis. This is exploratory surgery which looks inside the internal pelvic area. A tiny incision is made into the navel to view the pelvic region especially the ovaries and fallopian tubes. It is generally done under general anaesthesia.

Hysteroscopy

This procedure views directly inside the uterus. The main purpose is to see if the woman has fibroids or other reasons as to why she may not be able to carry a baby to full term. This is generally done with local anaesthetic.

Falloscopy

This is a new procedure that looks directly inside the fallopian tubes. It tries to diagnose any abnormalities of the tubes that might block sperm coming up or the egg coming down. This is done under general anaesthetic with a fibre optic telescope.

Many of these tests are extremely stressful. It is stressful if the tests are not normal but even if the results are normal it is frustrating as you still don't know what is wrong!

In my case I was advised to have the AMH(anti-mullerian hormone) test for ovarian reserve, all the blood tests for infections and hormone levels, HSG(Hysterosalpingogram). These all came back normal and one doctor suggested we go straight for IVF treatment. We decided against this initially as nothing had been found that was "wrong" as yet. We opted to try the IUI (intra uterine insemination) as it was less expensive, less invasive and no one had identified a specific reason for infertility (although there was a potential borderline issue with my husband's sperm count). We tried 3 attempts at IUI without success, but then became pregnant naturally 4 months later. I cannot explain why this happened but we were thrilled. We then went on to conceive naturally a further two times which were much easier than the first.

Would we have done anything differently? Probably not- in the end, we were very lucky. We did as much as we could to optimise our own health, took the advised tests and tried the IUI several times. If this failed, we would certainly have considered the IVF treatment as we had done all we could in every other area. We knew we wanted a baby and knew we had to try everything possible to make sure this happened. There were ups and downs and moments of stress, pain and doubt along the way. I am sure at times it created tension in our relationship with each other but this will happen in a situation where there is constant disappointment. We knew to expect this so were conscious to make time for each other, give support to each other and try to remain positive at all times.

But I wish to emphasise that every case is different. It can be very tough. Arm yourself with as much knowledge as possible and make sure the advice makes sense to you at the time given what you know about your own circumstances. Some of you will need to go straight for IVF if you have blocked fallopian tubes or your partner has minimal sperm. Some of you will be able to try less invasive methods and some of you will become pregnant naturally. If you are not sure, get a second opinion or a third opinion and read as much as you can about the procedures and the likely outcomes.

Resolving Infertility

There are only three ways to resolve infertility.

1) Optimise your chances of becoming pregnant naturally- correct timing of intercourse and clean up your diet and lifestyle

As you know by now this is achieved by being disciplined about charting so you can accurately time sex for the most fertile day. It is also achieved by both the man and the women improving their fertility by improving their health. Take vitamin and mineral supplements, give up smoking and drugs and reduce toxins, alcohol, caffeine and dairy. Some women may wish to try naturopathy or homeopathy.

2) Correct the underlying problem if one has been identified
3) Seek medical assistance in bypassing some of the steps required for reproduction. The next chapter discusses these options in detail.

Drug Therapy

If a problem has been identified with your hormones, drug therapy may be prescribed. Two of the most common ones are Clomid and Pergonal. Clomid is the least invasive of the two and it stimulates ovulation in women who are not ovulating or irregularly ovulating. In reality Clomid is often prescribed as routine even when the fertility problem is unknown. Clomid has the unfortunate side effect of drying up cervical fluid which is vital for sperm transport through the cervix so oestrogen is also prescribed to counteract its drying effects. The other is it can cause the second stage of the menstrual cycle to be too short thus preventing an egg from implanting in the uterus. You need to be aware of this and discuss these possibilities with your doctor. Clomid must be used appropriately and in the right circumstances i.e. if you do not ovulate- and you must be given advice about what to do to ensure there is sufficient cervical mucus present to enable conception to occur.

Progesterone is prescribed for women with short luteal phases which usually works very well allowing the fertilised egg enough time to implant into the uterine wall and then carry a baby to full term.

Pergonal is an extremely potent drug which is tried if Clomid does not work. Pergonal is usually used when the couple undergo IVF, GIFT or ZIFT(these procedures are discussed later). There are other hormonal drugs your doctor may prescribe if you have an imbalance of FSH and LH. Drugs can be tried to suppress ovulation in women with endometriosis. They decrease ovulation for six months then ask the woman to try to become pregnant again.

Surgery

Surgery can be performed to address polyps, scarring, endometriosis or fibroids. Sometimes surgery can be done via laser so it can be performed as an outpatient.

Four common female fertility problems

These are the four most common reasons responsible for female infertility. I am sure most of you will either have one of these or know someone with one of these.

1) Endometriosis
2) Polycystic ovarian syndrome
3) Luteinised unruptured follicle syndrome
4) Premature ovarian failure

Here are each of these in more detail:

1) Endometriosis

This is a surprisingly prevalent disorder where the normal endometrial tissue which lines the uterus begins to grow elsewhere in the body. The misplaced tissue may develop anywhere within the abdominal cavity growing in thick patches or within cysts in the ovary. The degree of pain is not consistent with the severity of the condition. It may cause excruciating pain but be small and contained or have minimal symptoms but spread extensively.

There are two types of treatment: hormonal or surgical.

The goal of hormone treatment is to stimulate pregnancy or the menopause which are the two natural conditions that inhibit the disease. Hormone treatment only works in mild cases.

Surgery on the other hand can remove adhesions, implants or blood filled cysts. Laparoscopy can drain fluid and remove small patches.

If you try all these methods and still have no success becoming pregnant, you will need to try IVF treatment.

2) Polycystic ovarian syndrome (PCOS)

PCOS may be the most prevalent hormonal disorder women have and one of the most common causes of endometriosis. Essentially what happens is the developing follicles that normally ovulate with each cycle stay trapped inside the ovary. After a while they swell with fluid and turn into cysts. If they are not treated they develop a hard shell making ovulation less likely. This is a hormonal problem caused by excess production of testosterone and excessive LH (luteinising hormone) and FSH (follicle stimulating hormone).

The cause is not understood but some evidence points to high blood insulin levels. PCOS results in obvious infertility, irregular cycles, excessive body and facial hair, male pattern hair loss, acne and obesity. There is also a higher risk of endometrial cancer. Unfortunately there is no known cure but treatments are improving. Treatment focuses on improving the sex hormone balance but also often includes treating the high insulin levels too.

3) Luteinized Unruptured Follicle Syndrome

Even if you have all the fertile signs, you still may not be ovulating. The luteal phase can be so short that it's not obviously a fertile cycle. Ultrasound may reveal that the ovum remains stuck in the luteinised follicle unable to pass through the wall. The only valid treatment in this case is IVF.

4) Premature ovarian failure (POF)

This is a case where the ovaries stop producing eggs a decade or so too early. On average a woman's ovaries should supply her with enough eggs until age 51 when the menopause begins. Unfortunately it is difficult to treat. Other health conditions are also associated with POF like osteoporosis, auto immune diseases, hypothyroidism and increased incidence of heart disease. By the age of 40, an estimated 1% of the population has POF. The symptoms are much more severe than occurs at normal age menopause. In many cases the cause of POF is unknown, sometimes it is attributable to auto immune diseases, chemotherapy, infection or genetic disorders.

There is no current established treatment for POF. There are an increasing number of women seeking donor eggs to enable them to conceive and have children. There are also studies being done at the moment experimenting with DHEA (discussed earlier) to increase spontaneous pregnancy rates and improve success rates of IVF treatment.

Make sure you are in control

Be careful that your team of fertility experts are finding the exact cause of your problem not just putting you on an assembly line of three months of Clomid, three months of IUI then 3 cycles of IVF. Once you seek fertility treatment do everything you can to nurture yourself and keep depression and anxiety at bay. Drug therapy and surgical treatment can offer hope and a solution to many couples struggling with infertility. Many of these treatments will resolve infertility and allow a successful pregnancy to occur. The many options for assisted reproduction using medical technologies is discussed in the next chapter. It is very important to make sure you feel in control at every step along the way. The "medicalisation" of infertility can lead to depression, loss of control and difficulties in relationships between couples.

It is important to keep talking- to each other, to experts, to friends and support groups. Simply burying your head in the sand will not help you reach a solution. There are a lot of people, support groups and counselling available to if you feel you would like to talk to someone, make sure you reach out.

Chapter 8 Assisted Reproduction: Decoded

Most people only think of IVF when they think of using technology to assist them to have a baby. Actually technology is so advanced now that there are many methods available for all sorts of conditions and stages of infertility. So do read this carefully and make sure you seek the treatment that is actually relevant for your exact symptoms and test results. Make sure you are not simply on a treadmill of moving from one procedure to the next.

The first three options are the least invasive: AI (artificial insemination), IUI (Intrauterine insemination) and FAST (fallopian sperm transfer system).

All place the sperm inside the woman at different places in her anatomy: either outside the cervix, within the uterus or within the fallopian tubes.

These technologies usually involve sperm washing to dramatically improve sperm motility. This is the process in which individual sperms are separated from the seminal fluid. The sperms are then used in intrauterine insemination (IUI) or in vitro fertilization (IVF). Sperm washing is a standard procedure used in infertility treatment

1) AI and IUI

These are the simplest and least technically complex of the assistive reproductive technologies.

Artificial insemination (AI) involves using a catheter to gently insert the man's sperm just outside or within the cervix whereas intrauterine insemination (IUI) involves placing the sperm directly into the uterus.

The sperm may be your partner's sperm or a donor. These days IUI is preferred over AI as it bypasses a number of infertility problems like low sperm count, poor motility, anti-sperm antibodies, poor quality cervical fluid, irregular cycles and endometriosis.

With AI, conception is most likely to occur if the sperm is deposited at the cervix on the last day of cervical wetness. However with IUI it is best if sperm is deposited in the hours immediately before and following ovulation which is best determined by a combination of charting, ovulation predictor kits and ultrasound.

2) FAST

Fallopian sperm transfer system (FAST) is one of the newest more promising AI technologies. It involves placing washed sperm directly into each of your fallopian tubes in the hours following drug induced ovulation as close to the egg as possible. By doing this fertilisation is likely to occur more quickly and easily.

3) IVF

IVF (in vitro fertilisation) is most commonly performed on women who have blocked fallopian tubes. It is also common where there is unexplained infertility, ovulation problems or male infertility. It involves monitoring the woman's ovulatory process, removing several eggs from the woman's ovaries, fertilising them with her partner's sperm in a petri dish then placing the two day old embryo back in her uterus. There is natural cycle IVF where a naturally released egg is collected or artificial cycle IVF where the ovaries are artificially stimulated and many eggs are collected.

The challenge with IVF is not fertilisation but implantation. Since the embryo must be transferred from the petri dish and implanted in the uterus earlier than would naturally occur (Remember natural fertilisation occurs in the fallopian tubes, not in the uterus. It then takes a few days to reach the uterus and implant).

4) GIFT

Gamete intra- fallopian transfer (GIFT) solves the implantation issue of IVF but it requires that the woman's fallopian tubes are open and the man has adequate sperm. As with IVF, the eggs are removed but the eggs and sperm are placed via a catheter in the fallopian tubes and left to fertilise on their own. This usually involves a minor surgical procedure and some pain for a few days. GIFT is more effective than IVF because placement of sperm and egg into the fallopian tubes rather than the uterus mimics the way a naturally fertilised egg would begin its journey to the uterus for successful implantation. Also it is the only assisted reproductive technology that is completely acceptable to the Roman Catholic Church.

5) ZIFT

Zygote intra fallopian transfer (ZIFT) is a procedure useful for where the woman's fallopian tubes are open but the man's sperm is marginal. The egg is fertilised in the petri dish and the resulting zygote is transferred to fallopian tubes and continues naturally down and implants.

As you can see IVF, GIFT and ZIFT all remove the eggs from the woman's ovaries. The difference's here are where fertilisation occurs- in or out of the body and where the egg and sperm are returned to the woman's body.

6) ICSI

Intracytoplasmic sperm injection (ICSI) is one of the more promising techniques for condition where the man's sperm count is low or has been unable to fertilise an egg in previous IVF attempts. The woman may have mild scarring from endometriosis or blocked tubes. A single sperm in injected into the ova via high tech instruments. After fertilisation is achieved the newly created embryo is placed in an incubator for 2-3 days before being placed in women's uterus.

7) **OT**

Ovum transfer (OT) is one of the most dramatic advances in fertility technology which allows a post-menopausal woman to carry and deliver a child. Using a petri dish, her partner's sperm are fertilised with a younger donor's eggs. The embryo is implanted back in her uterus.

It should be noted that until recently the option to freeze your eggs when you are younger was not possible because they were too fragile to withstand the procedure. Now improved technology will allow this to happen so women can have their own biological children when they are older and ready to become parents.

What procedures yield the best success rates?

It is very difficult to accurately compare different procedures and even the same procedures between different clinics. There are so many variables like the ages of both partners, respective health issues, diet, stress levels and so on. Also some of the clinics report "pregnancy rate" which often later miscarry when actually the statistic you really want is "healthy baby rate". Technology will continue to improve but success is never guaranteed and sometimes it does take several attempts to be successful.

It is generally accepted that GIFT and ZIFT have greater success rates than IVF. Many start with IVF as it is a simpler and cheaper option that can be performed on an outpatient basis.

Before you consider any of these options be aware that all involve a series of produces that may be both physically and emotionally uncomfortable. So make sure you discuss it with your medical team, go home and discuss it with your partner and make sure you are prepared. You will need to expect the unexpected - for example irrational emotions, extra stress, extra disappointment if one or two cycles fail. You will need to make a mental note to communicate even more with your partner during this time, to support each other more, be gentle with each other and allow each other to be a little crazy without taking it personally. Even though it may not be rational, the woman will be injecting herself with extra hormones which can play havoc with all her systems including emotional ones.

What actually happens in IVF, GIFT and ZIFT?

You will be prescribed a series of hormones which you will have to inject. The man's sperm are "washed" to improve motility. Then a dozen or so of the woman's eggs are aspirated from her artificially stimulated ovaries with a vaginal ultrasonically guided needle. Then depending on the procedure which I have outlined above, they will be fertilised (or not) then returned to her uterus or fallopian tubes.

There is also natural IVF where the woman does not inject hormones to artificially stimulate her ovaries. Her egg is collected from her natural cycle. This avoids many nasty potential side effects of the hormone injections one of which is excessive ovarian stimulation. Many cases are mild including vomiting, nausea and diarrhoea. But some cases can be severe and include chest pain, abdominal pain, shortness of breath and pleural effusion. This is why it must be very carefully medically monitored.

Mild IVF is a method where a small dose (30-40%) of ovarian stimulating drugs is used for a short duration. This aims to collect 2-7 healthy eggs instead of the standard 12-14 eggs. Mild IVF and natural IVF are cheaper and have fewer side effects than conventional IVF and there is evidence that birth weights of the babies are higher. Some clinics also offer natural cycle IVF in which no drugs are used at all. In the UK standard IVF is approximately £5,000; mild IVF is approximately £2,500 and natural IVF is approximately £1,500. In both mild IVF and natural cycle IVF the risk of ovarian hyper stimulation syndrome is drastically reduced. With mild IVF ovary stimulating drugs are given to a woman during her natural cycle whereas with conventional IVF, the practice is to induce an artificial menopause then kick start an artificial cycle.

When the eggs have reached maturity, the woman is given a HCG hormone injection and egg collection is done just prior to when the follicles would normally rupture. This HCG hormone injection can also induce ovarian hyper stimulation.

The eggs are retrieved by piercing the vaginal wall usually under general anaesthesia. Usually 10-30 eggs are removed. The eggs and the sperm are prepared and incubated to fertilise. In ICSI the egg is injected with the sperm then when the embryo become 6-8 cells it is transferred back into the woman's body.

How many eggs are transferred depends on the number of eggs available, the age of the woman and other health factors. In the UK, Australia, Canada and New Zealand, a maximum of two embryos are implanted back into the woman. In the UK though, if the woman is over 40 years old, three embryos may be returned. In the USA younger women may have multiple embryos returned depending on the individual fertility diagnosis.

Risk factors during IVF

One of the nasty side effects of the hormone injections is excessive ovarian stimulation. The symptoms are discussed above. It occurs in approximately 30% of patients. Mild cases can be treated with over the counter medications. In severe cases the woman will be hospitalised. This is why it must be very carefully medically monitored.

During the egg retrieval process, there's a small chance of bleeding, infection, and damage to surrounding structures like bowel and bladder (transvaginal ultrasound aspiration) as well as difficulty in breathing, chest infection, allergic reactions to medications, or nerve damage (laparoscopy).

IVF does not have increased risk of birth defects.

IVF Success Rates

Clinics may measure success by pregnancy rate or live birth rate.

Here are some statistics from 2009 USA national rate:

Technology is improving all the time and success rates also keep improving.

Age	<35	35-37	38-40	41-42

Pregnancy Rate	47.6	38.9	30.1	20.5
Live Birth Rate	41.4	31.7	22.3	12.6

There is also a difference using a live sperm versus donor frozen sperm.

Look at these numbers:

	Fresh donor egg embryos	**Thawed donor egg embryos**
Live birth rate	55.1	33.8

Stress and IVF

A Swedish study in 2005 found that psychological stress during an IVF cycle may not affect the outcome. However the experience of IVF can result in stress that leads to depression. The alternative to IVF for many couples may be infertility which can also lead to stress and depression.

Other factors that affect outcome of IVF

- Smoking in both men and women decreases success rates
- Excessive alcohol and caffeine decreases success rates
- Excessive body weight (BMI over 27) decreases success rates
- IVF success is significantly improved in women who maintain good humour and a positive attitude.

Summary

There are some cases where IVF does not work and some couples have to face the reality of infertility. If this happens expect your emotions to go through the various stages of grief which can take 3-4 years to deal with. You will mourn the children you will never have. Living with involuntary childlessness can wreck your sex life and cause you to reject anything that has family connotations like 4 x 4 car, kids' parties, living near schools. You will need to keep talking with people, develop new goals and interests but get professional help if you need it.

Do not underestimate the seriousness of infertility. It is a real physical and emotional shock to the system and you need to deal with and cope with your emotions. Don't think you "should" be coping better. It is major trauma and may take a long time to come to terms with.

First Test Tube Baby and the Future

The first successful birth of a "test tube baby" was Louise Brown in 1978 from a Cambridgeshire clinic in the UK. It was a natural cycle IVF and the physiologist who developed the treatment was awarded the Nobel Prize in Physiology or Medicine in 2010. In 2004 Louise got married and Dr Edwards attended her wedding. In 2006 she gave birth naturally to her own son.

IVF is now 35 years old and has produced more than 5 million babies. In 1978 it was viewed on with suspicion and clinics got hate mail and threats. It was expensive, costing around £3000 then when the national yearly income was just £6000. Women had to stay in hospital for 3 weeks. Now women are seen as day patients and it is much more accepted. The emotional, physical and mental health outcome for these children born from assisted reproductive technologies has been studied. The results show that in general born of parents who have been through an enormous amount of pain, anguish and expense to have them, that they have much lower incidence of problems at all levels than one would expect in the normal population. There is evidence to show they are more cared about and become much happier, contributing people.

There has been a report (Kate Brian, The Guardian newspaper 12 July, 2013) in July 2013 from Belgium doctors speaking at a conference in London that the cost of IVF could soon be cut from thousands of pounds to £170 due to new technologies they have developed. They said 12 children had already been born this way. As to the details- they have not yet been revealed to the general public but watch this space.

Where will we be in another 35 years?

Chapter 9 Yay! Early signs of pregnancy. OMG! What now?

Once you do get a positive test and confirm you are indeed pregnant, there will be a few weeks of bliss, just you and your partner keeping a special secret between you. Then a few weeks later the first horrid symptoms of the first trimester may commence. You will leave the weird and complicated world of conception and move to the weird and wonderful world of pregnancy. Be warned it is not suddenly all a bed of roses! Some women are fine and breeze through it but they are the minority.

Most women feel sickly nausea and extreme fatigue. Unfortunately this fatigue does not go away even with 9-10 hours' sleep which you will need to be getting. Early pregnancy can feel like having a bad flu for several months. Apparently this fatigue is caused by your uterus making the placenta that will support your baby. This takes a lot of nutrients away from you and saps your energy. Continue to eat as well as you can during pregnancy, exercise gently and go to bed early.

Obviously you will be charting your temperature so you will know before anyone else or any predictor kit that you are pregnant. You will have noticed your 18 days of raised temperatures.

You will also notice:

- Tender breasts and nipples
- Nausea
- Fatigue
- Excessive urination
- Implantation spotting (light brownish bleeding 8-12 days after ovulation).

How much value do Pregnancy tests offer?

You will be charting anyway- right? So you will notice 18 days of high temperatures. You can confirm with a home pregnancy test which is a urine test looking for the presence of the pregnancy hormone-HCG (human chorionic gonadotrophin). Sometimes you will get a false positive or a false negative missing the fact you are actually pregnant.

Most embryos don't implant until day 8-10 post ovulation. So don't bother testing until day 13 or so. It depends on the length of your luteal phase. Testing before day 12 can give you a negative result for three reasons even if you are actually pregnant:

1) The embryo implants late to the womb

2) You tested later in the day when your urine is more diluted

3) The test is not sensitive enough.

There is another problem with testing early. Many pregnancies miscarry in the first 4 weeks.

Across all ages the figure for pregnancies that miscarry is around 25%! So you might find out you are pregnant but only to find you get your period late. This is not a false positive - it is a loss. Sometimes it is better not to know.

On average women first start to feel pregnancy symptoms about 20 days after ovulation, the home test can detect it a few days earlier.

It is safe to travel in your first trimester but you will need to eat frequently and sleep just as much and speak to your doctor. You will not be able to take medication like sleeping pills or pain killers.

After that it will be a constant period of change as you observe your body shape changing, telling everyone, picking names, doing up the nursery, and fending off interested strangers who feel it is their right to touch your tummy!

And of course there are all the horror stories other parents drop on you, like you won't sleep again until they are 12 years old, the screaming, the tantrums and the teething but most new parents find these complaints are over exaggerated. Yes of course there is work involved but manage things early, instil discipline before the baby appoints them self the boss, communicate with each other about how best to manage situations and put up a united front between you and you will be fine. They are only small for a short time, then day care, then preschool, then suddenly you find yourself at their college graduation.

C section vs. natural birth

A Caesarean section (C-section) is a surgical procedure in which one or more incisions are made through a mother's abdomen and uterus to deliver the baby. A Caesarean section is usually performed when a vaginal delivery would put the baby's or mother's life or health at risk; although in recent times it has also been performed upon request for births that could otherwise have been natural.

In recent years, the rate has increased worldwide. It has risen to a record level of 46% in China, 33% in the United States, in Italy the rate is 40%, while in the Nordic countries it is only 14%. Doctors maintain that elective caesarean can be harmful to the foetus without benefit to the mother, and have established strict guidelines for non-medically indicated caesarean before 39 weeks.

The reasons for the rapid rise may be several. Some argue the cost of C section is higher, so the surgeons are quick to recommend it for pure financial gain. There is some thought also that a quick scheduled C section is more efficient for the medical team than a prolonged labour. There is also the increase in doctors being sued for complications with the birthing process so if there is any hint of a complication, they will recommend C section.

Others have found that some women may have lost confidence in their ability to cope with pain and elect for C- section hoping it will be less painful and traumatic.

Indications for C –section

It is worth remembering that there are fewer complications with operations performed during daylight hours than emergencies performed at night. So discuss carefully with your doctors probabilities of C- section and take into account, your health, your pelvis size, and the babies estimated birth weight. These are the typical indications for recommending C-section:

- Prolonged labour
- Foetal distress
- Cord prolapsed
- Increased blood pressure-mother or baby
- Increased heart rate – mother or baby
- Abnormal presentation e.g. breech

Risks for the mother

C -section is no light matter- it is major abdominal surgery. The UK National Health Service gives death rates among C- section three times as high as natural birth. Of course the results are a little skewed as high risk situations do require C- sections however it is a reminder that a C- section is a serious procedure and all the risks need to be considered carefully.

Other risks include incisional hernias, wound infections and severe blood loss. Mothers also experience higher risk of post natal depression after C- section compared with vaginal delivery.

Risks for the child

- Higher infant mortality risk: In C-sections performed with no indicated risk (singleton at full term in a head-down position), the risk of death in the first 28 days of life has been cited as 1.77 per 1,000 live births among women who had C-sections, compared to 0.62 per 1,000 for women who delivered vaginally.
- Wet lung is also a known complication: Retention of fluid in the lungs can occur if not expelled by the pressure of contractions
- There is the potential for early delivery and complications due to early delivery if the due-date calculation is inaccurate.

Recovery

A C-section is major abdominal surgery and takes much longer to recover from than vaginal birth. Typically, the recovery time depends on the patient and her pain tolerance and inflammation levels. Doctors do recommend abstention from strenuous work- lifting >10lbs (4.5 kg); running, walking up stairs, driving or athletics for up to six weeks and a waiting period of 18 months before attempting to conceive another child.

With vaginal birth, the women will be sore in the genital area for up to 3 months depending on tears and episiotomies during the birth. They may find sexual intercourse extremely painful for three months after the birth. There may also be significant back pain depending on trauma on the spine and coccyx during the birth. If you breastfeed, this will act as a contraception until you cease.

Ensure you do your pelvic floor exercises to restore your vaginal tone which drops at least 50%. So there may be incontinence sneezing and coughing in the early days until you do your strengthening work. There should be no long term deficit.

Chapter 10 Dealing with miscarriages

Miscarriages are surprisingly common. One in three pregnancies do not make it to 20 weeks (a loss after 20 weeks is considered a still birth). After six or seven weeks when a foetal heart beat can be seen in ultrasound about 15% of pregnancies still miscarry. The risk does increase with age. The father's advancing age is correlated with increased incidence too. Most miscarriages occur in first twelve weeks which is why most couples wait until then to announce the news to family and friends. Amazingly all the organs have already been formed by then and can be seen on ultrasound. So it does feel like a real little person, and you will have to be gentle with yourself and allow yourself to grieve.

If you are miscarrying on a reoccurring basis, all the high tech procedures discussed above won't help you as you ARE able to achieve pregnancy but the problem is keeping the embryo viable. As men and women progress into their thirties, miscarriages do become more common. As you already know, charting can play a massive role in understanding and diagnosing this problem (18 days of high temperatures followed by a sudden drop in temperature and eventual bleeding).

When you seek help from the doctor, you will need to ensure you get help for miscarriage not in actually becoming pregnant.

Also remember to keep things in perspective. If you have one miscarriage, the majority of women (87%) do go on to have healthy pregnancies and healthy babies afterwards.

What can cause miscarriage?

Infections

A bad cold or flu is not likely to harm your foetus but malaria, chlamydia, mycoplasma and toxoplasmosis may. Antibiotics are used to treat infections and some doctors prescribe it routinely as it is safe for mother and baby and may help prevent miscarriages in general.

Certain viruses are dangerous during pregnancy such as rubella, herpes, mumps measles and hepatitis A and B. If you are planning pregnancy make sure you are up to date with all your inoculations.

Hormonal problems

An abnormal luteal phase is the most common hormonal reason for miscarriage. As I discussed already for a fertilised egg to implant and mature the corpus luteum must maintain the latter part of the cycle for at least 10 days. Then it must live long enough for the placenta to take over the function of providing nutrition for the embryo. The corpus luteum should live 10 weeks beyond conception so if you miscarry before that the doctor will suspect corpus luteum deficiency. The doctor may prescribe progesterone to help address this problem.

Uterine abnormalities

Some women have a weak cervix which tends to dilate before the foetus is full term. In these cases sometimes a stitch in the cervix will help solve this problem. Other women are born with congenital defects of the uterus which means the baby can't grow big enough before the cervix dilates. These women will need surgery. Some women (about 40%) have fibroids. They are not usually a problem unless they are fast growing or cause severe bleeding.

Antibodies

Some mothers produce antibodies that reject's her own foetus. Blood tests will determine this. Your doctor will prescribe anti-clotting drugs, immunoglobulins or anti-inflammatory drugs. Some doctors may prescribe low dose aspirin or blood thinners like heparin.

Certain medical disorders such as uncontrolled diabetes, high blood pressure or heart disease also may predispose women to miscarriage. Make sure you talk to your doctor about making your health as good as possible before attempting to become pregnant again.

How to know if you are having a miscarriage

Spotting is very common in early pregnancy. You may notice a little bit of brown blood. However if you see red blood that is more than just spotting, it is more likely to be a sign of miscarriage. Most of the time doctors cannot do anything to stop a first trimester miscarriage once it has begun.

Other warning signs of miscarriage include headaches, cramping, dizziness, excessive vomiting and nausea, pelvic pain and falling temperatures.

If you were more than six weeks along in your pregnancy, you should see your doctor to make sure you miscarried completely. If not, dilation and curettage (D and C) may be required to clear the uterus. This is a procedure which dilates the cervix and surgically removes the contents of the uterus by scraping and scooping (cutterage).

Can I do anything to prevent the risk of miscarriage?

You should cut your risk of miscarriage by taking prenatal vitamins (both men and women), no smoking, cutting down on caffeine and alcohol, eating well and having sex just before ovulation (rather than the day of ovulation) as the egg is more likely to be healthy if fertilised right away. Remember nature makes the final call. Eggs can be damaged, sperm can be faulty, and the first cell fusion is simply a miracle.

Sometimes the DNA is faulty, sometimes there are natural chromosomal errors, sometimes when the cells divide something goes wrong. Even if you have done everything right and the sperm and egg find each other, there can be a problem at fertilisation, implantation or at many stages along the way. Doctors have found this may happen 60% of the time. It is a tenuous time with a lot that can go wrong which is completely beyond your control.

Even if you did everything right, a miscarriage still sometimes happens. It is no one's fault. Even after two losses, women do go on to have successful pregnancies. When you miscarry you will be grieving. Allow yourself time to adjust and come to terms with it. Be gentle with yourself. It may take you six months to a year to cope. It is always traumatic and the loss is generally felt worse the longer the pregnancy has continued.

Many women are surprised at their own reaction if it happens to them. Jacqueline wrote in to me "I never thought I would feel as emotional about it but I couldn't talk about it without crying for months."

Sarah said "The worst thing was telling my two year old boy that he was not going to have a little brother or sister now"

The hardest things will be other people's reactions and platitudes. What about your partner's reaction? Depending on how he deals with loss, his reaction may be the one that drives you right over the edge!! Remember everyone copes differently. The most important thing is to acknowledge this is a difficult time and to make extra effort to communicate often and openly.

How soon can we try again?

If the loss happened in the first six weeks of the pregnancy, you can start trying again immediately.

If it happened in the first trimester it is best to leave it one cycle then you may start trying again. If you required a D and C, your doctor will advise you but generally it is advised to wait three months for the lining of the uterus to build up again but also to allow you to emotionally deal with the miscarriage.

Chapter 11: What if it all goes right?

You can do this, stay positive, communicate, focus on the outcome - remember a lovely, helpless little baby who will grow, change and provide you with a lot of heart ache but also make you burst with pride. Even if you have struggled with infertility for several years, follow these guidelines as best you can. For many of you making a few lifestyle changes will help you fall pregnant naturally in the next few months. For others who do need medical assistance, you still need to be getting your body into the best health possible to ensure you have the best chance of the procedures working effectively. You will be able to approach your doctors and fertility experts with knowledge and intelligent questions rather than be led aimlessly in a state of confusion and helplessness.

I cannot promise every reader a successful pregnancy from this book, nor would you expect me to but I am sure you are a lot more informed, able to put yourself in the best position possible to enable a successful pregnancy to happen, and are more informed about assisted reproductive technologies available and which one is most likely to help you.

Of course there will be a few sacrifices in eating well, quitting smoking, cutting your bottle of wine a night to just one glass(or none at all), but remember when you have kids there will be a whole load more sacrifices to come! So it is good preparation. Remember this when you are doing the boring routine of charting your temperatures, in the stress of making sure you arrange intercourse on the "correct" day, when you are sitting in doctors waiting rooms, when you are being prodded, poked and scanned, when you are having your bodily fluids rushed off to be taken off to labs for analysis.

Remember to try to keep it light hearted and fun. Remain optimistic and remember to communicate with each other. You are a team, working together, towards the same goal. Keep visualising success, your healthy, happy baby. Keep visualising your healthy body, growing more and more radiant throughout your pregnancy. Keep optimistic, keep breathing and keep focused. Do not give up!

It WILL be worth it...

I have spoken a lot about all the things that can go wrong, potential problems and how to resolve them. For most of you this will result in a happy, bouncy, little baby- then your life will never be the same again.

In the meantime, if you and your partner are struggling with the stress, with understanding the process and most of all with your emotions in dealing with it "not happening" right now, do not let the magnitude of the task at hand overwhelm you. Remember focus on one step at a time and do not stop until each step is done.

Try to keep it all in perspective. Focus on what you CAN do right now and simply do it. There is a lot in your control, get your sleep, take your vitamins, cut back on all the toxins, breathe, communicate with your partner all the time and remain close and happy.

Try to enjoy the time you have together now as when you have the baby, you will have precious little time to yourself. Travel, do some trips, relax but for now please focus on your calendar, your charting and make darn sure you are timing intercourse for the most fertile two days a cycle.

Best wishes for your every success- and do get in contact with your success stories (and the names of your babies), I love hearing from you,

Jessica

@pregnancybible1

I really hope you enjoyed this book and got some clarity on the steps you need to take to maximise your chances of becoming pregnant and what steps to take if it is not happening.

If so, please spare one minute and leave me a review. I would really appreciate it as it makes all the difference.

Useful Websites

www.fertilityuk.org

www.ivf.com

www.obgyn.net

www.mum.org

www.createhealth.org

References

Bigelow, J.L, D.B.Dunson et al (2004) "Mucus observations in the fertile window: a better predictor of conception than timing of intercourse." Hum Reprod 19(4): 889-92

Dean, Cat; Sizer, Anya.(2010) Fertile Thinking. Infinite Ideas Limited, Oxford, UK.

Dunson D.B.,C.R. Winberg et al (2001). "Assessing human fertility using several markers of ovulation."Stat Med 20(6): 965-78

Encyclopaedia of alternative medicine 2005: Journal Therapy

Gray, R.H.,J.L. Simpson et al.(1998) "Sex ratio associated with timing of insemination and length of the follicular phase in planned and unplanned pregnancies during use of natural family planning." Hum Reprod 13(5): 1397-400

Hassan, MAM and Killick SR (2003). Effect of male age on fertility: Evidence for decline in male fertility with increasing age. Fertility and sterility, 79, 1520-1527.

Heffner, LJ (2004). Advance maternal age-how old is too old? New England Journal of Medicine, 351 1927-1930.

Hilgers, T.W. and A.J. Bailey (1980). "Natural family planning II. Basal body temperature and estimated time of ovulation" Obstet Gynecol 55(3): 333-9

How to Get Pregnant fast. Essential secrets for impatient couples trying to conceive. Tress Bowen 2012

Katz D.F.(1991) "Human cervical mucus: research update" Am J Obstet Gynecol 10(6): 223-228

Lauersen, Niels H, MD. and Colette Bouchez. Getting Pregnant: What You Need To Know Right Now. New York, Simon and Schuster, 2000.

Medical News: "Sperm Swim Singly After Vitamin C Therapy." Journal of American Medical Association 249 (May 27, 1983): 2747-2751

Overstreet, James W, David F Katz and Ashley I Yudin. "Cervical Mucus and Sperm Transportation in Reproduction" Seminars in Perinatology 15 (April 1991): 149-155.

Pyper, C.M. and J. Knight (2001) "Fertility awareness methods of family planning: The physiological background, methodology and effectiveness of fertility awareness methods." The Journal of Family Planning and Reproductive Health Care 27(2):103-110.

Ruebinoff, Benjamin, E. And Joseph G Schenker "New Advances in Sex Preselection" Fertility and Sterility 66 (September 1996) 343-350

Sachs, Judith. What Women Can Do About Chronic Endometriosis. New York. Dell Medical Library, 1991.

Scher, Jonathan, M.D. Preventing Miscarriage. New York. Harper Collins, 1991.

Taking Charge of Your Fertility. The definitive guide to pregnancy achievement, natural birth control and reproductive health. Toni Weschler 2003

Twenge PhD; Jean. M The Impatient Woman's Guide To Getting Pregnant

Wilcox, A.J.; C.R.Weinberg et al (1995) "Timing of sexual intercourse in relation to ovulation. Effects on the probability of conception survival of the pregnancy and sex of the baby." N Engl J Med 333(23):1517-21

Winston, R. A child against all odds, Bantan Press, 2006

www.ingramcontent.com/pod-product-compliance
Lightning Source LLC
Chambersburg PA
CBHW071808170526
45167CB00003B/1228